The **POWER**
of
COMMUNITY

CrossFit
and The Force of Human Connection

Allison Wenglin Belger, PsyD

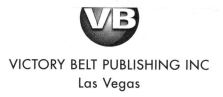

VICTORY BELT PUBLISHING INC
Las Vegas

First Published in 2012 by Victory Belt Publishing.

ISBN 13: 978-1-936608-73-7

Printed in The United States.

In thinking about the power of community and the impact of group support, what I have come to understand is that you may not know what has been missing until you discover it, and you can't imagine the possibilities until they begin to unfold.

Vulnerability is uncomfortable. Taking risks is uncomfortable. Pushing our bodies to physical extremes is uncomfortable. Being emotionally engaged is sometimes uncomfortable. And yet, each experience allows us to discover something more about ourselves than we knew before. Each encounter encourages growth, insight into ourselves, and a greater appreciation for those who have helped us along the way. The more we engage with others and the more we are open to others, the more likely we are to persevere and succeed in times of stress. Communities can do wonders for people, and these affinity groups don't need to be formal or structured; they simply need to provide support, ongoing contact, and a sharing of experiences.

Table of Contents

Acknowledgments

I'm told that writing a book is a great accomplishment. As with all achievements in my life, this one could not have happened without the support and help of many people.

Above all, the content of this book exists because of the individuals who are part of the TJ's Gym community. It is their joy, suffering, friendship, enthusiasm, and willingness to share of themselves that inspired me to document a phenomenon of connection that is alive and well. I am also thankful to others, once strangers, who generously shared their stories during interviews so that my readers would be able to feel the power of community through their experiences.

Thank you to Erich Krauss at Victory Belt Publishing for believing in my ideas and working with me all the way.

Thank you to my dear friend and teammate, Lisa Rendic, for being the kind of friend one can only dream of meeting as an adult, with quality of connection overcoming the lack of a shared childhood. You inspire, challenge, support, and encourage daily.

My mother, Barbara Wenglin, a reference librarian who taught me how to write, made darn sure this book was a good one. I am beyond grateful for her attention to detail, passion for grammar, and absolute determination to get me to do the best job I could. Thank you, Mom, for putting your heart, as well as your mind, into this book. And to my Dad who holds us all together.

A project like this that consumes its author also consumes her loved ones. I love to write, and it comes relatively easily for me. Still, my journey in writing this book meant hours and hours at my computer. My daughters are gems for supporting the venture and understanding that I was up to something big. I can only hope that this exposure to seeing a project through will benefit them as they grow. I feel sure that it will. Our children are great barometers for what is worthwhile in life.

My endlessly patient husband, TJ, has put up with every last bit of this all-encompassing endeavor and has helped immeasurably with the trajectory of the book. His creative approach and generation of ideas made the outcome far better than it otherwise would have been. TJ is the man at the helm of our community—a giver, a provider, a leader in the best sense of the word. He is a wonder of a person who deserves a world of recognition.

Prologue

I have a confession. I used to read magazines while I exercised. I used to wear headphones at the gym. Normally quite social and relationship-oriented, I was driven to avoid eye contact with others. I wasn't there to socialize. I was there to work out and get some happy juices flowing. I would tell myself that my routine was exactly what I needed to stay in shape and counteract my well-developed sweet tooth. I didn't need more friends. I just needed the machines. I would glide almost unconsciously on the elliptical machine, or race the stairs on the Stairmaster, holding on for dear life. I would throw in the occasional biceps curl and triceps extension and call it a day. I would leave as stealthily as I came so nobody would be tempted to start up a conversation.

How ironic then, that in 1996 I would meet my future husband, TJ, at a gym in San Francisco. He was a personal trainer and I was given three free training sessions when I joined. My usual guard was up when we met but over time I relented and our flirtation grew into a lasting relationship. Our gym courtship still makes me smile when I think about it.

When TJ and I left the city a few years later and moved to suburban Marin County, he was in the process of looking for space to open his own personal training studio. I was working toward a doctorate in psychology in Berkeley and needed a gym nearby that would be convenient before school hours. I found a typical membership gym and became, as I had many times before, a reluctant member of such an establishment.

At this gym, the cardio machines were upstairs on a balcony overlooking the workout floor below, and my standard form of entertainment involved sensory input through ears and eyes. The headphones I wore played a mix from my early post-college years, and my psychologist-in-training eyes took in the nuances of the social interactions I watched unravel below. While I didn't know any of the people and couldn't hear what they said, their outfits, body language, and facial expressions were fodder enough to create life stories for them all. It was as though my music was the soundtrack for screenplays of each imaginary life playing out in the theater of my little analytical mind.

September 11, 2001. I was on a machine on that balcony, people-watching as the early birds punched their workout clocks below. I noticed in my peripheral vision that there was a crowd of people gathering near a television screen. Clearly there was something going on in the news. I have vague memories of seeing flashes of fire and smoke coming out of buildings, but I didn't dare leave my perch on the Stairmaster to find out what was going on. At some point, though, I gathered that something terrible was happening in New York City, and I was shaken. I grabbed my belongings and bolted home, racing to contact loved ones as so many of us did on that day. The last place I wanted to be was at a gym filled with strangers.

Life has changed significantly since that horrible day. I finished school, became a psychologist and a mom, and helped TJ open gyms of our own. As I reflect on the global changes that have occurred in our lives over the past ten years, I realize that were tragedy to strike now while I was at the gym I wouldn't race out so quickly. Of course my first response would be to ensure the safety of our children, but after that I would want to be surrounded by the warmth and camaraderie of my gym community. These are people who have become an extended family, with whom TJ and I have shared ups and downs, people who know our children and whose children we know. I no longer wear headphones when working out. I no longer avoid eye contact and I no longer pretend that an effective workout can be done while reading a magazine. My workout world has expanded to include community, which has made it both more effective and more enjoyable.

In a recent blog entry on our TJ's Gym website, TJ asked the question "How uncomfortable are you willing to get?" He was making a point akin to "there's no such thing as a free lunch," or the old exercise adage, "no pain, no gain," but from a psychological standpoint: positive change usually involves some degree of discomfort. If you want to be different or feel different or live differently, or if you simply want to get better at something, you need to be ready to be uncomfortable along the way. Based on my own experience as a gym goer and as a psychologist, it is far easier to be uncomfortable—to allow ourselves to be vulnerable and take risks—when we have the support of others along the way. We can do infinitely more for ourselves and for others when what we are doing is grounded in some kind of community.

The notion that people can accomplish more in groups or thrive with social support is not new, but my goal here is to relate the story of a powerful kind of community that is growing by the minute, every day, across the world. It is a community based on an exercise program founded in science, driven by data, and comprised of functional movements repeated throughout a lifetime. It is a group of people sharing insight into optimal nutrition and sleep practices, inspiring each other to achieve fitness levels once unimagined by its participants. It is a community dedicated to the health and wellness of its members, with a philanthropic edge to boot, as you'll see in the coming pages. It is the global community of CrossFit and our local version of it in our TJ's Gym affiliates.

This book is not designed as a marketing tool for CrossFit. The people at CrossFit headquarters had nothing to do with my initial idea to write this, nor did they have any input during the writing stage. My praise for CrossFit comes from my own experience, as a psychologist, an athlete, a coach, and an affiliate gym owner. The CrossFit community is thriving and growing at a time when community affiliations have decreased overall. I write about CrossFit from a psychosocial perspective because it is a unique program that exemplifies how a community can provide the fuel that powers our wellness as individuals.

We will hear stories of people like you and me whose lives have been improved in important and meaningful ways by their involvement with a CrossFit community. We will also hear of individuals who have drawn upon their passion for CrossFit to create other communities benefiting people in need. We will hear about how young adults with cancer, military wounded warriors, underprivileged at-risk youth, recovering addicts, and many others are benefiting from the generosity of people who have created support networks for them. We will hear about a pro-bono school exercise program and a thriving corporate community changing the lives of its employees for the better. Through these stories, we will begin to understand the human drive to bond with others and the importance of finding a safe place of connection. We will gain insight into the experience of vulnerability, of primal physicality, of risk-taking and discomfort, and how we can each tolerate more than we think, as long as we are supported along the way. This will lead to practical applications and conclusions for creating a better, healthier, more fulfilling life.

Throughout our discussion, "community" will be defined loosely as a group or groups of people with enhanced social connections who are mutually engaged in an activity, common interest, or pursuit. An important aspect of community, as discussed here, is that it provides social support, which results in both personal and public benefits.

Chapter 1

Background on Us

TJ and I met in 1996 at a 24-Hour Fitness gym in San Francisco. I had just finished my master's degree in learning disabilities at Northwestern University and had moved back to San Francisco, where I had lived after college, to start the next phase of my adult life. One of the first things I did after finding a place to live was join a gym. My new membership included three free private sessions with a personal trainer. Although I knew private training would not be part of my long-term exercise plans, I accepted the offer and showed up for my first appointment where I was greeted by TJ. We were both immediately interested in each other, though neither of us made that clear for months down the road.

We married in Lake Tahoe in July 2000 and moved out of San Francisco into suburban Marin County shortly thereafter. I was back in school pursuing my doctorate in psychology, and TJ had moved his personal training clientele to a smaller, private club that offered him greater autonomy, marking the first big step in his fitness career. Soon he was scoping out spaces for his own personal training gym and found just the right one within a mile of our home in San Rafael. The site we chose is approximately five thousand square feet, one portion of a larger building housing three businesses. We built ADA bathrooms, cordoned off a small room where Pilates and yoga classes would be held, and spruced up the rest of the space that would be the gym floor. By this time, I had completed my doctoral coursework and was two months away from defending my dissertation. I was five months pregnant when we opened Personal Fitness Institute of Marin in March of 2002.

During the final weeks of my pregnancy, with my title of "Dr." now official and forever sealed, and with my licensing internship on hold until after the baby was born, I spent many hours at the gym, walking on a treadmill or just hanging out to see if there was anything I could do to drum up business. I was in the midst of a break, preparing for motherhood after earning my degree. When a potential new client walked in, I would perk up and give them our pitch, explaining that we weren't a typical membership gym but offered, instead, a place where trainers could operate independently and clients would enjoy a pressure-free, scene-free place to work out with top-of-the-line equipment. Slowly we brought in new clientele. However, our business plan was not well constructed, and we soon realized that TJ's training income, though great for someone who didn't have to carry his overhead, was barely making a dent in our considerable expenses. We were still making ends meet with the help of family and bank loans, which, we were assured, was typical of a new business.

In August of 2002, our first daughter, Lyle Sadie, was born. Her entry into our world was as joyous and remarkable as most births, and we were on cloud nine. Soon we were in the thick of new parenting with the usual sleep deprivation and all-consuming focus on our new child. I was grateful that TJ worked so close to home, since there were times when I'd call him, driven to tears from hormones and lack of sleep, begging for an hour respite from mothering. Other times I would strap the baby in a carrier and walk over the hill to the gym, fulfilling my need for fresh air, exercise, and adult interaction in one fell swoop. As Lyle grew, I would take her in a stroller and have the hum of the treadmill sing her to sleep while I worked to reclaim my pre-baby body and get some endorphins flowing. The business trudged along, with new trainers popping in every so often, having heard about the friendly and hands-off management of the new gym. At one point we even introduced spinning classes, funded by one of TJ's clients who was convinced that we could make a killing with a spinning studio. We didn't.

During the time between the end of 2002 and the summer of 2007, life went something like this: I completed the 1,500 post-doctoral supervised hours required to become a psychologist; TJ's workload increased, but we still wondered how we would ever profit from the gym; I gave birth to our second daughter, Hollis Brooke; and I took a part-time psychology position working with children and adolescents in San Francisco. We hired our first and fabulous nanny to cover while I worked, which added to my sanity and gave me an identity outside of motherhood, but also ate into our profits. My work was fascinating and rewarding but also immensely taxing and stressful, and after a couple of years of commuting, I was ready for the chance to try being a mom with fewer career demands.

For his part, TJ still loved working with his personal training clients but realized there was only so much he could do to change their lives when he only worked with them for a few hours each week. My input about the mind-body connection would often cut through the heart of the client-trainer relationship. Indeed, it's a funny thing living with a psychologist: you get to hear all the no-bullshit stuff about what you and other people are up to. I would tell him things like, "When your client tells you she's not eating any crap but is still gaining weight, she's lying," or "That guy isn't going to stop canceling last-minute until he finds a way to get out of his abusive relationship with his partner." TJ listened and became even more driven to use his passion for fitness in ways that could transform the lives of his clients.

One day in the summer of 2007, a teenage client who was part of a group of homeschoolers TJ trained, burst into the gym with a newspaper article about the fantasy action film "300." He asked TJ how the actors in the film could have possibly become so ripped and lean and muscular in time for the film shoot and assumed that they must have taken steroids. TJ thought so too until he did a little research and found that the actors and extras in the film had been trained using a fitness program called CrossFit. This discovery would prove to be the beginning of the rest of our lives.

TJ read up on CrossFit on its website, an awe-inspiring assortment of articles, videos, pictures, and knowledge about fitness and nutrition, all available free. He began trying the workouts and though he immediately felt results, he kept it to himself for some time, not wanting to go public with the program until he was sure he knew what he was doing and had faith that it would work in the long term. He was quietly getting the crap kicked out of him with his workouts, modified as they were due to equipment constraints, limitations of what his body was ready to do, and lack of coaching. Combining Olympic weightlifting, gymnastics, cardiovascular training, kettlebells and more, CrossFit is difficult to take on without in-person guidance, despite its accessibility online. Still, TJ continued using the CrossFit program and knew he had found something special.

While on vacation visiting our families on the East coast in August 2007, TJ and I had one of those conversations that mark a significant change in a family's course. We decided that unless something drastic happened to change the gym's business model, there was no way it was going to support our family. I encouraged TJ to start networking with people who held positions of power in organizations, companies, and schools throughout the Bay Area. I reminded him that he possessed a number of qualities that would serve him well in any field, as long as he could work with people. He was a natural motivator and an approachable leader with all kinds of compassion, sensitivity, and level-headedness. Further, he had the work ethic and desire to match anyone in any workforce, and he would apply that wherever he landed. The conversation was difficult and somewhat depressing, as it seemed that TJ's dream of having his own gym might soon come to an end.

TJ returned to work after that vacation with fire in his belly and a secret mission to save the gym, believing that CrossFit would ultimately be the way to do it. He quickly approached his early morning training clients to see if they would be willing to forego their semi-private sessions and give group training a try. He explained that he had found a new way of training that was sure to lead to faster and better results, based on a group process that was shown to provide motivation and focus. He called the workouts "Metabolic Conditioning," not truly CrossFit workouts at the time, but derived from the research he had read about how one can actually make changes at the metabolic level. He borrowed from the CrossFit approach enough to utilize functional body movements, encouraging members to increase their intensity during workouts, a fundamental aspect of CrossFit. These classes quickly grew and TJ found himself emptying his pockets each evening of the cash he had collected from drop-ins that day.

By March of 2008, I had started doing certain portions of the new workouts that appealed to me. I jumped on boxes, swung kettlebells, and did strict pull-ups. I ran, squatted, and threw medicine balls. I liked the way these workouts made me feel, and I was no longer bored. TJ was onto something! He and some other trainers at our gym became CrossFit certified and TJ began researching the process of officially converting to a CrossFit gym. While on the CrossFit message board, he hooked up with John Burke, a guy from Los Angeles whose business partner was apparently doing amazingly

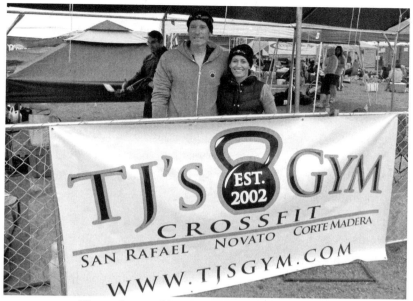

The author and her husband, TJ Belger, at the
2009 CrossFit Games in Aromas, CA.

well with his CrossFit gym, even though it was only about 1,000 square feet.

John encouraged TJ to come down to LA to talk with him and his partner, Andy Petranek, about how they ran their business. They called it a Business Apprenticeship Program, and TJ would be in the second cohort they'd ever trained. The cost for five days of business coaching and access to all of their systems would be five thousand dollars. Holy crap, I thought. Five thousand dollars! That's a lot of diapers and student loan payments. Looking toward the future, we bit the bullet, paid the money, flew down to LA with our girls in tow, and TJ learned how to make the transition from pockets full of singles to legitimate and regular credit-card transactions. He learned all sorts of other things as well, and when we returned from LA, we immediately implemented much of what we had heard. We became an official CrossFit affiliate, and our lives were about to change, as were the lives of so many people who have since crossed our paths.

This book is about the process of changing lives for the better. It is the story of how we were able to adopt a brilliant fitness program and make our version of it work for hundreds of people. It is a story of how psychology is intertwined with physiology, how nutrition goes hand in hand with exercise, how emotions fuel energy systems. It's about executing your first pull-up, attaining personal records in Olympic lifts, and learning gymnastic movements as an adult, all within a welcoming space that fosters these changes. It is about people reaching out to those less fortunate and providing opportunities for fellowship and support. Globally, it is about the human drive to connect with others and the inspiring ways in which these connections can bring about change. It is about the thriving worldwide phenomenon of CrossFit and how TJ's Gym fits within that larger sphere; this is a story about human relationships, personal growth, and the power of community.

Chapter 2

Background on CrossFit

Why do people work out? What drives the multibillion-dollar worldwide fitness industry? What makes individuals join one gym over another, choose one type of class over another, or purchase one type of home-gym equipment over another? What makes one person stick with an exercise program and another jump from one fad to the next? Why do people pay for gym memberships they never use? We know that exercise decreases our risk of obesity, heart disease, and other illnesses. We know that it activates endorphins in our endocrine system and affects our mood. We know that exercise burns calories and helps lower levels of bad cholesterol and that it can be a way to meet other people and connect on a social level.

Our doctors, our therapists, our coaches, our parents, and our teachers all tell us that regular exercise leads to happier and healthier lives. But exercise programs vary dramatically, and it can be difficult to navigate the world of fitness programs and products, gym memberships, training manuals, and gadgets, whose creators all claim to have found the golden ticket to the fountain of youth or the ideal body. Few programs are backed up by legitimate studies or robust data demonstrating their efficacy in producing practical, lasting benefits. All too many exercise crazes seem to disappear into oblivion just as quickly and dramatically as they appeared, leaving once-avid practitioners searching for the next best thing.

In the 1970s, a former collegiate gymnast from Santa Cruz, California, Greg Glassman, decided to put together what he thought would be an effective workout program that would lead to optimal levels of fitness. He recognized that fitness should involve some measure of applicability to everyday life, that such a program would include a wide range of physical activities, each of which would tax a human body system in different ways. He did not buy into the notion that a person who could run or bike or swim the farthest or the fastest was necessarily the fittest overall. He questioned conventional ideas about fitness and endeavored to create a fitness standard that would be broad and inclusive, rather than specialized and circumscribed. Through research and exposure to athletes, many of whom were military personnel and law enforcement officers whose jobs required a certain level of physical ability, Glassman redefined the notion of fitness and created a unique exercise program that would lead people to new levels of personal achievement and a higher level of general physical preparedness.

Glassman's concept of fitness demands capacity in ten general physical categories: cardiovascular/respiratory endurance, stamina, strength, flexibility, power, coordination, agility, balance, and accuracy. Capacity is measured within all three of the main metabolic energy pathways driving human action and movement: the phosphagen pathway characterized by a surge of activity lasting ten seconds or less (e.g., an explosive weightlifting effort); the glycolitic pathway, which dominates efforts lasting ten seconds to several minutes; and the oxidative pathway, primary in activities lasting beyond several minutes and as long as several hours (e.g., a marathon). Finally, Glassman's fitness requires the ability to perform rigorous physical tasks and various combinations of movements when unfamiliar demands and requirements are introduced. The idea is that the fittest individuals are well prepared for whatever life throws their way, whereas individuals with a more circumscribed fitness regimen have limited success outside a specific domain.

Imagine the world's fastest marathoner faced with the task of lifting a large log off his car after a storm. Likewise, think of the massive powerlifter, who also happens to be a police officer, trying to chase down a suspect. You get the idea: how can we train to develop a type of fitness that adapts to any situation, challenge, task, or demand, whether it's something we've done a thousand times or never before? How can we maximize the potential for good outcomes in real-life scenarios that demand physical abilities? How can we make ourselves more flexible and coordinated while also building our strength, power, speed, and endurance?

With science and experience to back him up, Glassman knew that a CrossFit program could provide the answer. Now a worldwide fitness phenomenon, CrossFit started as a grassroots effort in local garage gyms. The first CrossFit gym—or "box"—was located in Santa Cruz, where Glassman introduced his athletes to the idea that some combination of cardiovascular training, gymnastics movements, Olympic weightlifting, and powerlifting would lead to greater levels of fitness than any one of these modalities alone. He further believed that intensity and variety were keys to making changes in athletes at the metabolic level, as adaptation would quickly set in if those components were omitted. He also figured out that it was critical to make use of the phenomenon that human beings perform better in groups. Hired by local police departments and devoted to helping military personnel prepare for battle, Glassman made early inroads into these communities and continues to be active in both to this day.

In 2001, Glassman launched CrossFit.com, a website where followers could find a daily workout that would prescribe a series of movements they could follow at their convenience. They could also view instructional videos for each movement from Olympic weightlifting to gymnastics to cardiovascular exercise and could read about Glassman's approach to managing nutrition for optimal performance.

Over the years, CrossFit has expanded to include various certification seminars, with thousands of CrossFit affiliate gyms operating worldwide. These facilities vary dramatically in size, scope, style, and kind, but share in common the CrossFit methodology as their principal exercise program. They are not franchise locations; rather, affiliate owners pay a modest annual fee to use the CrossFit name and to market themselves as CrossFit facilities. After that, they are on their own to implement the program and operate their business as they choose. Each affiliate must have a unique registered owner, which prohibits a single entity from cornering the CrossFit market. Indeed, Glassman's vision includes competing CrossFit gyms on every corner. Customers abound, since he argues that his broad and inclusive program is applicable to all body types and fitness levels, famously stating in the *CrossFit Training Guide* that "the needs of Olympic athletes and our grandparents differ by degree not kind."[1] Despite the massive growth of CrossFit, what permeates its existence both online and in vivo, is a sense of community and social connectedness; this is, arguably, as essential to its efficacy and popularity as are the fitness tenets and methodologies to which it adheres.

When TJ and I converted our gym to a CrossFit affiliate in April 2008, we were pretty sure that CrossFit would enable us to grow our business while helping our client base become more physically fit. After all, conventional wisdom states that physical fitness and strength translate into higher levels of mental health and productivity, and who wouldn't want to serve that up in large doses? If we could make a living while making a difference in people's lives both physically and psychologically, that would be a wonderful thing. We imagined how the business might run, but looking back, we had no concept of the magnitude and power of the community we were on the verge of creating. Over the past three years, we have opened three more affiliates, two in partnership with colleagues and friends; we have expanded our membership to close to 1,000, ranging in age from four to eighty; we have sent athletes to compete at the worldwide CrossFit Games; and we have witnessed the internal and external transformations of many people whom we've had the privilege to call clients and friends. This book is as much their story as ours.

The following chapters will highlight the stories of a number of individuals whose lives have been significantly changed by their involvement in our gym community and by the strength they have gained through CrossFit. These are people who have overcome tragedy, who have made important health gains, maintained dramatic weight loss, and improved their mental outlook. You will also read about people who are creating a social network of support for others in need, promoting well-being and making lives better through their generosity of spirit and a strong sense of purpose.

We can all find ourselves in these stories. We share a drive to feel strong and secure, connected and supported, comfortable and capable in our bodies. We seek ways to achieve wellness and contentment in uncertain times, to approach the future with increased confidence and improved quality of life. We will demonstrate how communities provide the support to accomplish much more than we ever could on our own. Indeed, communities are a critical aspect of the human experience, as we will learn through the stories that follow.

Chapter 3

The Importance of Community

"The community has a way of making a person feel important, which has the ability to save a life."
-Olivia Smith, age seventeen, TJ's Gym member

My brother Jason was a corporate lawyer in New York City in the 1990s. Having graduated from fancy institutions of higher learning, he landed a position at one of Manhattan's most prestigious law firms. He was on the fast track to partnership when he became interested in studying the Talmud, a compilation of Jewish legal texts that have been interpreted by scholars for centuries. As his interest intensified and the spiritual aspect of his life expanded, he eventually left his career as an attorney, moved to Israel, and pursued his studies with fervor.

Today my brother is a Rabbi in Israel, married to an American-born woman who shares his worldview, with six children and possibly more to come. In many ways Jason and I live very different lives: we live in opposite time zones halfway across the world. Though we are both parents and spouses and wish for all good things to happen to our families, our cultures, beliefs, passions, drives, and daily routines differ in dramatic ways. I initially had a hard time accepting his transformation from hot shot lawyer living a secular life in Manhattan, to bearded, ultra-Orthodox Jew whose life bore little resemblance to the one we knew growing up in suburban New York in the 1970s and '80s. Now I realize how my understanding of my brother's life has evolved over time, as I have come to create a community of my own.

My own assumptions were transformed when TJ and I had our first child. As so many new moms are, I was bewildered by many aspects of parenting, but perhaps the most disquieting for me was the experience of isolation that often overwhelmed the more blissful moments of this new role. Beyond the wonder and joy of it all, there were the moments of feeling separated from the rest of the world, trapped by the sleep-eat-poop routine of this newborn, so helpless, needy, and demanding, but also the most beloved and treasured little being one could possibly imagine. After my mother's month-long visit had ended and the last of the baby gifts had been opened, I felt disconnected from adult life and unwittingly delegated to a new identity that was unfamiliar and uncomfortable at times. I longed to feel connected to something larger during this time of extreme connectedness within the mother-child dyad.

My doctoral dissertation, which I had completed during my pregnancy, drew heavily on the work of Donald Winnicott, a British psychiatrist who wrote about the mother-infant relationship. He describes this as being so inherently intertwined that the infant has no psychological experience of separateness until it has the capacity to realize that it is not actually one with its mother. The emergence into psychological separateness is managed by the healthy mother whose "maternal environment"—marked initially by an unwavering attunement to the infant's every need—establishes a foundation of security and dependency in the infant who can then become prepared for separation. When all goes well, this is a beautiful thing, allowing us a gentle experience of psychological separateness, all at an unconscious level.[2] I found that I was part of this process, both intellectually as a student of Winnicott, and unconsciously as a new mother. Much as the baby must become able to manage delays in gratification, the mother I had become also had to accept my own need for independence. In retrospect, I appreciate the health that comes with a well-titrated emergence from that "maternal environment" and the accompanying readiness for interactions outside of the mother-infant relationship.

Joining a mom's group was clearly an attempt at separation, but meeting once a week with other new moms and talking about diapering and nursing schedules only provided so much relief. In fact, there were times when being around a group of new mothers who once were lawyers and physicians and politicians but could now only seem to talk about nursing bras made the yearning for a larger community even more intense than when I was alone with the baby. It's not that life wasn't magical then; it certainly was, and the joys far outweighed the struggles. But our culture has a way of separating parents from nonparents and mothers from the women they once were. The first exposure to this separation can be curious and even unsettling, if not overwhelming.

Over time, much as I have disagreed with my brother's and sister-in-law's choices, what I have come to appreciate about their lifestyle is the emphasis on community. Rabbis and students gather in study groups to maximize learning. Certain daily prayers require a "minyan" or quorum of participants. The synagogue becomes a center of communal life. Mothers have many babies and are often nursing one while diapering another. Families live in defined neighborhoods where the older children watch over the younger ones and what happens to one family is experienced by another. Celebrations and tragic events are shared across family lines. The Sabbath table is a warm and welcoming communal gathering place in the home. Babysitters come from within the family or neighboring homes; the community raises its children. Teachers are mothers and mothers are teachers. There is a sense of connectedness and a reassurance that one's children are looked after and cared for by the extended community.

The proverb, "It takes a village to raise a child," adopted by Hillary Clinton for her 1996 book, is actually quite in line with my brother's community and with much of what I am exploring in this book. Clinton's work, *It Takes a Village,* outlines her ideas about the importance of the people and influences beyond immediate family who have a significant and lasting impact on the development of our children. Her book was a call to action for building a society committed to the collective rearing and watching over our nation's young people:

> *Children exist in the world as well as in the family. From the moment they are born, they depend on a host of other "grown-ups"—grandparents, neighbors, teachers, ministers, employers, political leaders, and untold others who touch their lives directly and indirectly. Adults police their streets, monitor the quality of their food, air, and water, produce the programs that appear on their televisions, run the businesses that employ their parents, and write laws that protect them. Each of us plays a part in every child's life: It takes a village to raise a child.*[3]

No matter one's political leanings, Clinton's message has its place. My brother's community in Israel reflects many of her tenets. While aspects of this kind of connectedness may be seen in secular modern suburban America, finding that experience of communal support is more challenging with friends and families scattered across the country and around the world. Today's neighborhoods are less connected by walkways and outdoor space, or places for public gathering. Technology has had an impact too, permeating our relationships and allowing for immediate, constant contact while at the same time promoting separation and distance. We may have created and found sources of community within social networks and relationships, but we have to work harder to cultivate genuine human connection than we might in a culture founded on shared norms and belief systems.

While my brother's life choice is based in large part on faith and ritual, the importance of community in his world is what resonates for me. Francis Fukuyama, an American philosopher and political economist, discusses how religious affiliation can be seen as an expression of the human desire for connectedness. His thesis describes connection not just to a hierarchical structure or higher power but also connection to other people who share norms and morals:

Instead of community arising as a byproduct of rigid belief, people will come to religion because of their desire for community. In other words, people will return to religion not necessarily because they accept the truth of revelation but precisely because the absence of community and the transience of social ties in the secular world make them hungry for ritual and cultural tradition. They will help the poor or their neighbors not necessarily because doctrine tells them they must but rather because they want to serve their communities and find that faith-based organizations are the most effective means of doing so. They will repeat ancient prayers and re-enact age-old rituals not because they believe that they were handed down by God but rather because they want their children to have the proper values, and because they want to enjoy the comfort and the sense of shared experience that ritual brings. ... Religion becomes a source of ritual in a society that has been stripped bare of ceremony, and thus is a reasonable extension of the natural desire for social relatedness with which all human beings are born.[4]

In retrospect, it makes sense that the foundation of what would become a powerful form of connectedness and community for me and TJ had its roots in our early parenting years. There was no conscious plan or blueprint, and while we did not affiliate with a religious community, as my brother did, or with any other clearly defined network, what evolved from our days of nursing babies and abiding by nap schedules, of hiring babysitters to gain access to the outside world in our need to connect beyond our nuclear unit, was the development of a thriving gym community that is both large and powerful on the one hand, and intimate and sensitive on the other.

As an outgrowth of the larger, worldwide CrossFit community, our TJ's Gym community has provided immeasurable benefits to us and to hundreds of others over the past three years. While I know that our community is a particularly strong one, both in numbers and connectivity, I realize that we are not alone in our approach. In fact, there are many other CrossFit communities around the world whose members are reaping the benefits of social support and whose lives are far better because of their involvement in the program. CrossFit communities worldwide are thriving examples of how people are finding ways to connect with each other and maximize life experiences that include productivity, health and wellness, and a sense of purpose in a world in which group affiliations have declined dramatically. CrossFit both attracts and inspires people who understand and appreciate the power of group support and a shared commitment to positive change.

Chapter 4

The Benefits of Community

The power and benefits of community and social support have been widely recognized by writers and researchers across academic fields from a variety of intellectual landscapes, including sociology, psychology, behavioral sciences, anthropology, history, epidemiology, and more. We know that communities can provide the kind of social support and connectedness that foster a myriad of positive outcomes in people's lives. The term *social capital* has been used by many to capture how social networks have the capacity to increase productivity and lead to desired outcomes for their members. In his book, *Bowling Alone*, political scientist Robert Putnam explains that social capital is the mechanism through which social networks can impact individuals and societies. According to Putnam,

Social capital refers to connections among individuals—social networks and the norms of reciprocity and trustworthiness that arise from them. In that sense social capital is closely related to "civic virtue." The difference is that "social capital" calls attention to the fact that civic virtue is most powerful when embedded in a dense network of reciprocal social relations. A society of many virtuous but isolated individuals is not necessarily rich in social capital.[5]

Putnam further explains that the earliest known use of the term *social capital* was by of L.J. Hanifan in 1916, advocating for community support of the schools for the betterment of public education in West Virginia. Hanifan's social capital meant

goodwill, fellowship, mutual sympathy and social intercourse among a group of individuals and families who make up a social unit. ... [T]he individual is helpless socially, if left entirely to himself. If he comes into contact with his neighbor, and they with other neighbors, there will be an accumulation of social capital, which may immediately satisfy his social needs and which may bear a social potentiality sufficient to the substantial improvement of living conditions in the whole community. The community as a whole will benefit by the cooperation of all its parts, while the individual will find in his associations the advantages of the help, the sympathy, and the fellowship of his neighbors.[6]

Communities, as mentioned earlier, are defined as groups of people with enhanced social connections mutually engaged in an activity or common interest or pursuit. They provide the kind of social support that has been shown to have both individual and public or group benefits. Social networks create and make use of social capital and are thus means for people to experience positive connections and generate action within a culture.

Putnam describes a number of areas in which social capital has positive effects on our lives. First, he explains how the welfare of our children, from a psychological and educational perspective, is impacted by social capital; "trust, networks, and norms of reciprocity within a child's family, school, peer group, and larger community have wide-ranging effects on the child's opportunities and choices and, hence, on his behavior and development."[7] According to Putnam, good things tend to happen to children immersed in enhanced social support networks, while bad things tend to happen to children lacking in such networks. Then Putnam shows us how social capital leads to safer and more productive neighborhoods, how it not only counteracts the negative effects of poverty and disadvantage, but also leads to economic growth and prosperity. Finally, and most relevant to my own interests, Putnam reviews the impressive body of research, including the work of Emile Durkheim, indicating that the extent of one's social connectedness greatly impacts one's physical and psychological well-being.

Durkheim was a French sociologist instrumental in establishing sociology as an academic discipline. In his seminal work, *Suicide*, first published in 1897, Durkheim suggested that suicide rates were linked to the extent to which people were integrated into a societal group and their behaviors were regulated by societal forces. The societal groups could be religious, domestic, or political; it wasn't the content of the connection that was important, but rather "the degree of integration of the social groups of which the individual forms a part."[8] His idea was that the more connected an individual is to a group, and the more that group influences the individual's behavior, the less likely that individual will succumb to suicidal tendencies:

> *When society is strongly integrated, it holds individuals under its control, considers them at its service and thus forbids them*

to dispose willfully of themselves. Accordingly, it opposes their evading their duties to it through death. ... For they cling to life more resolutely when belonging to a group they love, so as not to betray interests they put before their own. The bond that unites them with the common cause attaches them to life and the lofty goal they envisage prevents their feeling personal troubles so deeply. There is, in short, in a cohesive and animated society a constant interchange of ideas and feelings from all to each and each to all, something like a mutual moral support, which instead of throwing the individual on his own resources, leads him to share in the collective energy and supports his own when exhausted.[9]

Since the publication of *Suicide*, numerous authors and researchers have cited Durkheim's work, analyzed his findings and theories, and positioned themselves based on what he suggested. His idea that suicide is related to a lack of social connectedness supports my research. Most of us know from our own life experience, or anecdotally through others, that the support of friends and social networks plays a role in lifting our mood when times are tough. Having a place to be, a group to be with, an activity to do with others, can all prove therapeutic when we feel lonely or down.

Lisa Berkman is a social epidemiologist and a leading researcher on the role of social networks and support in the physical health and wellness of individuals. Over the years, she and her colleagues have conducted numerous studies exploring the association between social integration and mortality rates and disease course. Berkman and her collaborators have found evidence that socially-isolated individuals have higher mortality rates than those who are socially-integrated[10] and numerous other researchers have reached similar findings. Further studies have shown a correlation between social integration, susceptibility to disease, and recovery from illness.[11] Levels of social support are also implicated in resiliency to stress and trauma: the degree of social support in one's life has a significant impact on how one manages in the face of serious stress and potentially traumatic experiences.[12]

There seem to be a number of possible explanations for how social integration improves health and wellness. These include greater access to health care and the accompanying lower levels of stress, as well as a greater likelihood that healthy behaviors and routines will be reinforced through social connections. Biological explanations are also supported by a rigorous body of research, indicating that social connectedness can have an effect at the cellular level.[13] Putnam provides an excellent overview of the research on the health benefits of social connection, demonstrating that social connectedness can help us live healthier and longer lives. Putnam advises:

> *The bottom line from this multitude of studies: As a rough rule of thumb, if you belong to no groups but decide to join one, you cut your risk of dying over the next year in* **half** *[emphasis in original]. If you smoke and belong to no groups, it's a toss-up whether you should stop smoking or start joining.*[14]

How about doing both—stop smoking *and* start joining? If social connectedness and social capital have been shown to have positive and lasting impacts on the physical and psychological health of individuals, CrossFit communities have the potential to take on a particularly powerful role. Organized around an exercise program that has clear, observable, and measurable physiological benefits, and founded upon a system designed to increase human work capacity and physical wellness, these social networks offer a leg up in terms of their opportunity to make positive changes in people's lives. CrossFit's emphasis on sound nutrition and a healthy lifestyle gives it more power to change lives for the better. In other words, both the *content* of CrossFit (the program, itself) and the *process* of how the CrossFit methodology is transmitted (the group setting with shared fitness goals) will contribute independently to positive outcomes, making the combined effect that much more powerful.

We see from Berkman's work that communities have clear and positive impacts on members' health and well-being even when the social support of a network is not based on fitness or wellness. Throw in a sophisticated, scientifically-derived, and data-driven road map to functional fitness as the core norm and value of the group and the combined effect is as intense as the workouts. Research by Kasisomayajula Viswanath and colleagues in 2006 at the Harvard School of Public Health showed how community ties can affect one's absorption and recall of health information.[15] Their study, which focused on information about cardiovascular disease but can likely be generalized to other health content, found that community membership had a positive effect on information recall and an even greater effect when subjects were members of organizations providing health information.

Applied to CrossFit communities, this makes perfect sense— membership in a group whose goal is to spread information about exercise, nutrition, health, and wellness will positively affect members' retention of such information. According to Viswanath, people become "primed" to take in and recall health information through their community, and when such content is disseminated within that community, the effect can be exponentially beneficial.

When people join a CrossFit gym, they usually hope to do something good for themselves, with a goal of improving their general fitness. While they may have heard about the camaraderie that is often part of the gym culture, the initial and most powerful draw is the possibility for change in their lives. This focus goes hand in hand with the emergence of community; bonds often develop and strengthen in organic ways, even when members are initially self-focused. As researcher Mark Smith explains: "Self-interest may bring people together, but in interaction something else emerges."[16]

In this vein, Zygmunt Bauman, a Polish sociologist who was driven out of Poland by the Communist purges, recognized that people can do more in groups than they can on their own:

*We are all interdependent in this fast globalizing world of ours, and due to this interdependence none of us can be the master of our fate on our own. There are tasks which each individual confronts but which cannot be tackled and dealt with individually. Whatever separates us and prompts us to keep our distance from each other, to draw boundaries and build barricades, makes the handling of such tasks yet more difficult. We all need to gain control over the conditions under which we struggle with the challenges of life—but for most of us such control can be gained only **collectively** [emphasis in original].*[17]

In an interview at the 2011 CrossFit Games, founder Greg Glassman was asked to speak about the community component of CrossFit. Coach Glassman explained how human performance improves "immediately" when workouts are completed in groups, or even when completed in the presence of a single other person. Beyond the mere results of a workout, there is a greater lesson to be learned from this phenomenon:

We all give more of ourselves in the presence of others. Always. Always. ... There's a coming face to face with the reality that you get only back what you give, and people extend themselves places they've never been before ... there's a critical life lesson there. Super critical. It's one of the most important things I can teach someone—to dig deep and give of themselves beyond what they would have assumed they had the capacity to.[18]

Arbella's Story

Arbella is part of what has consistently been the largest demographic in our TJ's Gym circle. Marin County is filled with young families. A typical trajectory involves college graduates moving to San Francisco, attracted by the accessibility and culture of the city, the temperate climate, and the proximity to mountains and the ocean. It is a city filled with outdoor enthusiasts, and fitness is a common pursuit. When these San Francisco folks get married and start a family, they often move north to Marin County, drawn to the excellent public schools and a quieter life. The TJ's Gym community is home to many such couples.

In her early forties, mother of two young children, Arbella had been a member at a larger gym in Marin for years. Once a marathon runner and triathlete, Arbella no longer had the time to train for such events, and her gym visits were only meant to salvage some of the fitness of her pre-baby world. Over time, Arbella became bored with her gym routine and couldn't fathom another day of running on a treadmill. A friend told her about a place called TJ's Gym. Arbella was intrigued by her introductory session with TJ and was surprised by the time he took to explain his CrossFit program. "We met, we

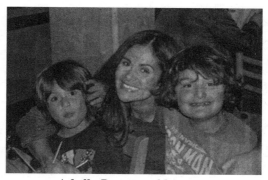

Arbella Parrot and her sons.

talked … I, exercised. It was hard … but I was hooked." With this taste of a new kind of workout and an experience she'd never had at other gyms, Arbella signed up for classes and became a regular at our San Rafael location. She remembers an initial period when members were on an honor system with payments and would just bring in cash or a check when they thought they were due. As for developing friendships, she recalls, "I would chat with people before class. As there was only one location at the time, you knew where everyone would be. It was a lovely feeling. I never did anything with anyone outside of TJ's, but it didn't matter. Everyone was happy to see you when they did."

She was also excited about the nutrition component of the program and was doing her best to make use of the education offered at the gym to get her nutrition in line with her pursuit of optimal physical performance and overall health. And then there were the actual CrossFit workouts, themselves: "There was no time to send emails, change songs on your iPod, chat with others … you barely had time to breathe! And I loved it." By August of 2008, Arbella was coming three times a week, splitting time between the two locations near her home. After many months of experiencing gains in her fitness, tracking her workouts, posting on the gym discussion board, and attending special gym events, Arbella was fully immersed in the TJ's community.

Then one day in the spring of 2009, Arbella received some shocking news. A routine mammogram had revealed a lesion in her breast. Further testing confirmed that she had breast cancer. As Arbella began sharing her devastating news with close friends and family, she knew she would have to include me and TJ. She called me aside one day before class and explained what was going on. We talked through the workout, through tears and hugs, and we parted that day embracing hope and promising that we'd figure out whatever plan would work best for her. While I couldn't offer one single bit of medical advice or reassure her that everything would be okay, what

I could promise with every ounce of my being was that there would be hundreds of people behind her in this fight of her life. In typical fashion, the TJ's Gym community stepped right up to help.

Margie, having been the recipient of this kind of help during a time of family crisis, spearheaded the meal delivery schedule for Arbella and her family. I was in charge of making sure her boys were well-stocked with DVDs, as the hours late in the day were typically the most exhausting for Arbella. We took walks, often talking about a non-FDA-approved technique she was using to salvage her amazing hair—a long, thick, black mane for which Arbella was known. Other TJ's Gym members accompanied her on hikes and walks, as this was the level of rigor Arbella could tolerate through her treatment. She received flowers, gifts, and cards—all sent by gym members, many of whom she had never met. There were trips to our Corte Madera gym, a short walk from her home that provided a place of solace and comfort. Still, these visits sometimes left Arbella in tears as they forced her to reckon with the fact that for others life goes on, while her own life was in a holding pattern of terror and fear. She longed for the workouts and that feeling in her body, but just couldn't handle the effort now. As she watched others in the gym, Arbella held fast to her goal of getting back to training once her treatments were over.

Thankfully, Arbella endured it all with grace and fortitude, and her hair did not fall out, an added bonus. She returned to her workouts as soon as her body allowed, and she again immersed herself in the gym community, both in classes and on our discussion board. In October 2010, Arbella received a huge welcome and standing ovation when we held a "Burpees for Breast Cancer" event at our Novato location. We raised over $5,000 that evening, in honor of Arbella and the other courageous men and women within our community who have struggled with cancer.

We can easily lose sight of how fortunate we are to have our health. As I sit here today writing this chapter, I feel deeply indebted to Arbella, whose perseverance, strength and grace in the face of fear and pain have inspired us all. One of the most joyous and moving evenings I've spent in the past decade was at a beautiful party for Arbella on the year anniversary of her diagnosis. Surrounded by family and friends, many of whom were TJ's Gymers, Arbella joined us as we raised our glasses in a toast to her health and long life.

Chapter 5

We Are Driven to Connect with Others

I am not overstating things when I say that the support I got from the TJ's community during the time around my brother's accident changed my life.

-Margie, age forty-three, TJ's Gym member

Human beings are social animals. Born dependent on nurturers for every aspect of our survival, we are wired to attach to, and connect with, other people from the very beginnings of our lives. While psychologists with varied theoretical perspectives differ greatly in their beliefs regarding our sources of motivation for connection, from Freudians who talk about biological drives for instinctual satisfaction, to followers of Bowlby who say we are motivated to form relational attachments with those who care for us, most would agree that we are social creatures who reach out however we can to make connections with other human beings. Beyond the level of intimate relationships with our caregivers and close family members, there is also the question of whether or not we are driven toward connectedness at a communal or societal level. Based on my research and experience, I firmly believe that we are.

Despite the egocentricity of young toddlers, we see year after year, in preschool after preschool, the coming together of youngsters as they develop a mini-community of learners and social cooperators. As children move on to grade school and find connections with classmates, they tend to gravitate toward activities with friends, such as softball or choir. Although these groups are often facilitated by adults, it is the children who cooperate and make the connections with clear intent and obvious results, one of which is wanting more of the same. We see social networks and connections develop in high school clubs across America; in the fraternities and sororities on college campuses; and in groups of lawyers, bankers, doctors, teachers, firefighters, and police officers whose jobs bring them together. These communities can be fostered aggressively and with purpose, or by default and more organically. They can be more or less organized and structured, with greater or lesser degrees of social capital, but their existence is clear. Scientist, journalist, and professor, Matt Ridley, eloquently summarizes how the human social drive to cooperate and come together is part of what makes our species unique:

Humans have social instincts. They come into the world equipped with predispositions to learn how to cooperate, to discriminate the trustworthy from the treacherous, to commit themselves to be trustworthy, to earn good reputations, to exchange goods and information, and to divide labour. ... Far from being a universal feature of animal life ... this instinctive cooperativeness is the very hallmark of humanity and what sets us apart from other animals.[19]

Similarly, in his work, *The Great Disruption* (1999), in which he discusses the decline of social harmony in the 1960s and '70s, Fukuyama endorses the notion that our very nature as people inclines us to engage with others at some kind of societal level. He states that *human beings are by nature social creatures, whose most basic drives and instincts lead them to create moral rules that bind them together into communities. ... There is an increasing body of evidence coming out of the life sciences that the standard social-science model is inadequate, and that human beings are born with pre-existing cognitive structures and age-specific capabilities for learning that lead them naturally into society. There is, in other words, such a thing as human nature.*[20]

Relationships with family members meet our drive for connection to a certain extent. However, we also seek a connection to a larger group; extra-familial bonds propel us forward as we find satisfaction in the greater community. L.J. Hanifan recognized this back in 1916: "Even the association of the members of one's own family fails to satisfy that desire which every normal individual has of being with his fellows, of being a part of a larger group than the family."[21] From Elizabeth Frazer we hear of the power of our communal drive, how it enables us to overcome relational challenges and other potential threats to the ties that bind: "… [T]he aspiration to community is an aspiration to a kind of connectedness that transcends the mundane and concrete tangle of social relationships."[22]

My Personal Journey through Communities

I was born in Kansas City, Missouri. At the time of my birth, my father was a medical resident at the University of Kansas. Our family would live in two other states before landing in a suburb thirty minutes north of New York City in time for my first-grade school year. Growing up in Scarsdale, New York, was pleasant and replete with opportunities. My brother and I were encouraged to try all sorts of activities, from learning to play musical instruments, to trying out for sports teams, to attending sleep-away camp in the summer. For me, some of these activities stuck (sports), while others didn't (flute and violin). I tended to be more interested in group activities and team sports and less interested in individual pursuits.

As I reflect now on the experiences that have remained with me and shaped the person I am today, they have in common a social network of communities comprised of my peers—fellow students, athletes, and teens. In looking back, the connections that molded me most, beyond interactions with immediate family, were those that occurred within a group of individuals doing what I was doing or to whom I related in some meaningful way.

My earliest run-ins with team sports and group competitions came during color war at camp. The simple psychology of having half the camp population wear green and half wear white had profound effects on campers' perceptions of group belonging. There was something magical about wearing your colors and immediately sharing a bond with others, simply because you were sporting the team garb. This bond was strengthened, of course, by team contests in which we all engaged, but the external trappings of group identity were surprisingly powerful.

Longer-lasting and more involved team experiences came throughout my childhood and adolescence as I participated on athletic teams rotating with the seasons. With soccer and field hockey as my two high school varsity sports, I experienced the joy of participating in communities of athletes connected around a healthy activity made richer by competitive outlets played in the great outdoors. Over the years, our parents became part of these team communities, as did our coaches and their families. We connected across otherwise powerful social divides in the world of adolescence—more pretty or less pretty, Catholic or Jewish, AP student or remedial—categories that mattered little during team practices, bus rides to games, or in the heat of battle.

It is no secret that participation in team sports can do wonders for teen athletes, especially affecting girls' self-esteem and confidence. Beyond this, in our current context, one can argue that the positive outcomes from girls' sports have everything to do with the social support and connectedness athletes enjoy. My own experience with team sports continued during college, where I was a member of the varsity soccer team. Attending Dartmouth, a once all-male bastion, I was encouraged as a freshman to reach out to groups of women, and it helped that I was naturally inclined to do so. While joining a sorority seemed strange and artificial to me in some ways, the possibility of connecting with another group at a time when I was far from home, without the familiar support of my high school buddies, was extremely inviting. Being part of that group offered me opportunities to make new friends, participate in a variety of activities, and reach out to the wider community in philanthropic ways.

Post-college years in America can be fraught with uncertainty, and mine were no exception. I moved out to California to be near my college boyfriend who had grown up in the Bay Area. I was thousands of miles from home, living on the opposite coast from my family. My first job was as an intern teacher at a private school for boys in San Francisco. My social life involved mostly friends from college who had also trekked west. As I think back to those relatively turbulent years in my early twenties, I wonder if part of the emotional uncertainty had something to do with the lack of community in my life. Sure there were the typical struggles to choose a career path, fall in love, seek out life passions, settle on a geographical location. But these all might have been mitigated had I been more connected with a community of some kind. I had friends—lots of them, in fact: some were running partners, some movie friends, some shared my addiction to peanut butter frozen yogurt. But for the first time in my life, I was not a part of a larger, cohesive community based upon a mutual engagement or common goal, and never before had I felt so unsure of myself or my path. Even adolescence, with its internal chaos and ever-present uncertainty, questioning, and the occasional bout of angst, wasn't nearly as unsettling for me as those early post-college years.

During my years of adult self-analysis and psychotherapy, I've tended to think of this period of uncertainty as a result of leaving behind the structure of academic and family life and becoming an independent adult—no small task. However, I am now quite convinced that the lack of community in my life at that time of transition had a profound impact on my state of mind. Perhaps somewhere in the recesses of my psyche I recognized this at the time, and I was thus eventually driven to adventures that would provide in spades and with great intensity a social connectedness and community experience. This would become the central life-changing formula that I would draw upon throughout my future and while building our CrossFit community.

When I was growing up, Scarsdale was not known for producing rugged naturalists or hardcore adventurers. An affluent suburb of New York, Scarsdale was more famous for churning out Ivy League students and future professional success stories, captains of industry and leaders in academia. While intensity was part of the lifestyle, it was mostly directed toward performance—on standardized tests, in AP classes, in the importance of reading great literature, and in team sports. We had to immerse ourselves in extracurricular activities—to be well-rounded, but with a focus on one or two in order to stand out.

The holy grail of getting into a "good" college was pretty clearly laid out by the time we entered high school. We were encouraged to do interesting and inspiring things with our summers, in part, so that we could talk about them in our college essays and at campus interviews. We were privy to many luxuries. Life was hard in some ways (pressures to succeed), but easy in others (we had a whole lot of resources at our disposal and life was good). While I was always known for being an athlete and a tough competitor, I also liked my creature comforts. I never strayed far from home without my hairdryer, for example. This continued through college, where, despite being at a school known for its access to the outdoors and an emphasis on experiences in nature, I enjoyed the New Hampshire setting mostly from the comfort of my dorm room and got my outdoor fix during soccer practices, training runs, and watching other sporting events.

So it came as a bit of a surprise to those closest to me when I decided to go on an Outward Bound backpacking trip in the Eastern Sierras two years after graduating from college. While many of my friends from Dartmouth had done such trips during high school or college, the thought had never crossed my mind until I was twenty-two years old and, apparently, ready at last to experience the challenges of life in the wilderness. I can remember trying to convince my father with a great sense of urgency that I needed to go on this trip –with his financial assistance—even though I would be out in the mountains during Yom Kippur, the holiest day of the year in the Jewish calendar. This was one of those moments when parents try to exert the same influence on their adult children as they once did, forgetting all the intervening months and years when their kids were doing things other than what they, as parents, would have wished. In this case, my father needed to find an acceptable way to allow me to go off and not observe the holiday in traditional ways.

As I negotiated with my father, I told him that I would not be ignoring the point of the holiday at all: my understanding of Yom Kippur was to check in with yourself, take stock of the previous year, and make improvements in your relationships, in your behavior, and in your life so that you would be a better person in the year to come. How fitting, then, to be heading out into the wilderness, stripped of the superficial trappings of life as I knew it, and forced to reckon with what I had inside in order to survive the elements and contribute to a meaningful group experience. How much closer could I get to God than being high in the mountains away from the material comforts and distractions of civilization? My parents conceded, and off I went on this spiritual and physical backpacking adventure.

Always introspective and analytical, I was attracted to Outward Bound's emphasis on gaining insight into oneself when out in the wilderness. It turns out that much about being in the backcountry appealed to me, especially the bare-bones, stripped-down, raw and gritty aspects of surviving in the outdoors. The physicality of it all suited me well—I've always had that ability to dig down and push through physical discomfort, whether during a long run or hard soccer practice in the rain. In fact, it's clear that there's something I crave about pushing myself to physical limits, a characteristic I'm sure I share with most serious CrossFitters. When I was out in the Sierras as a twenty-two-year-old explorer, CrossFit as we know it didn't exist, but I was gaining access to parts of me that would be reawakened years later during workouts and gatherings with other athletes at CrossFit events. And my hairdryer was nowhere to be found!

I gained great insight into group dynamics during this Outward Bound experience. One of the things that happened when this collection of vastly different individuals ventured out into the woods, reliant on each other for survival, is that we were forced to find common ground. Human nature seemed to compel us to discover aspects in each other that allowed for connection, while overlooking personality traits that would force us apart under different circumstances. By the end of our twenty-two days in the beautiful Sierras, our group had become cohesive—to a point. The reality was that our different personalities could not overcome all friction in such a short time, but there was certainly a feeling of community, a camaraderie built upon an intense shared adventure, and, for me, an understanding that this was something I wanted to experience again.

Looking back, I can appreciate the mix of appealing elements in this personal outdoor challenge: the escape from the routine of my life at home; the crisp, dry air against the granite of the Sierras; the connections I had developed with my trip leaders and fellow adventurers; and the physical feeling I had in my body, chiseled as it had become from twenty-two days of backpacking. The combination of these factors drew me back to the wilderness four months later, this time to a destination even further away, in the remote region of Patagonia.

Need Food, but I'll Take a Hug

～

January 17, 1994. The Northridge earthquake hit the Los Angeles area, reaching a magnitude of 6.7 with massive ground acceleration that led to great loss and destruction, including numerous deaths. My brother was living in L.A. at the time, and he was unreachable by phone as my plane took off from JFK airport en route to the outback of southern Chile. I would spend the next seventy-five days with no possibility of contact with the outside world. Now, as a parent, when I think back to that rainy New York morning, I have great empathy for my parents and the anxiety they must have experienced, worried about one kid directly in harm's way and the other embarking on a dicey, risky journey. (We later learned that brother Jason was shaken but safe.)

My parents had agreed to subsidize a semester with the National Outdoor Leadership School (NOLS), during which I would trek by foot across glaciers and hills and kayak through the waters of Patagonia. I had signed on to the most extreme trip I could find, testing my mettle and resolve and forcing me to see if I really had what it takes to deal with this heightened challenge. It's one thing to fall in love with life outdoors when you're in the Sierra Nevada mountain range where it is sunny and dry most of the time, and where you are surrounded by awe-inspiring rustic beauty. Seventy-five days in Patagonia, known for its horizontal rains and fierce terrain, is an entirely different story—as I would soon find out.

The trip from New York to the fjords of southern Chile was a long one, especially since I didn't know anyone en route. When I finally arrived at the NOLS base, I was tired but ready for my next adventure. I had never kayaked before, so the prospect of living out of a kayak for over a month was daunting. And while I was confident in my newfound love of backpacking, I had also been warned about the rough terrain we would encounter and was introduced to something called bushwhacking. The first step was to meet our group leaders and begin the process of making connections that would develop over the course of the next seventy-five days.

The unfolding of group dynamics in the face of extreme conditions can be intriguing, life-saving, frustrating, gratifying, puzzling, and downright maddening at times. As the group encounters challenging terrain, extreme weather conditions, unfamiliar physical demands and a lack of any creature comforts, the human relations element takes on a drama of its own. There were great conversations shared in calm moments—paddling with fellow kayakers, swapping stories about how we had ended up in Patagonia—but there was also quibbling over who did more work when setting up camp or who ate more from the limited food supply. There were the inspirational moments of people overcoming fears and pushing through their perceived physical limits to make it from one camp to the next. And then there were the moments of depletion, of sheer exhaustion and ultimate discomfort. We went to sleep night after night soaked from head to toe, our fancy waterproof gear having succumbed to the relentless horizontal rains. I will never forget the sensation of taking off my wet clothes and layering them over my shivering body as I got into my sleeping bag so that the body heat I generated during sleep would dry my garments by morning. It never quite worked, but at least they were warm and wet, instead of cold and wet like our boots.

While I have lost touch with my comrades in Patagonia, my relationships with them mattered a great deal during those seventy-five days. In the circumstances described, if you can't make connections and work in cohesion, you are doomed. You need each other—to help clamp a backpack, start a fire, cook a meal, treat water, find a place to lay your head. You need a helping hand with an ice axe or an ear to listen when the going gets tough and you feel defeated. You need to feel connected when you long for home and miss your loved ones. And, sometimes, when bad weather prevents the float plane from dropping food at a lake as planned, you need a shoulder to cry on. With no food, unremitting rain and little fire, the days by this lake were truly miserable. I remember opening a watermelon-flavored Jolly Rancher candy and sucking every last bit of life from it, as though it were some sort of miraculous, life-saving nectar from home. We were on day five without food, and the weather showed no sign of abating. The hike out of camp would take days and the terrain was horrific—which we already knew because we had hiked in the same way.

To call what developed among a group of strangers during this intense trip a community might be a misnomer. However, there was certainly something deeply communal and connected about the experience, which has stuck with me all these years. I recall feeling that I would not be able to keep going without the support of the others, and I also knew that they could not do it without me. That reciprocity of dependency was both reassuring and frightening.

I include this excerpt from my Patagonia story as an example of how people can confront physical and psychological discomfort when they come together with a common goal or shared experience. When significant physical and emotional demands are present, group interactions are intensified. Vulnerability is uncomfortable. Taking risks is uncomfortable. Pushing our bodies to physical extremes is uncomfortable. Being emotionally engaged is sometimes uncomfortable. And yet, these experiences allow us to gain insight into ourselves. Each encounter encourages personal growth and a greater appreciation for those who have helped us along the way. The fact that those around us are going through similar physical, mental, and emotional challenges, supporting us as we support them, allows us to push ourselves in new ways. The more we engage with others and the more we are open to others, the more likely we are to persevere and succeed in times of duress. As we have seen, communities can do wonders for people, and these affinity groups don't need to be formal or structured—they simply need to provide support, ongoing contact, and shared experiences.

Lisa Berkman and her colleagues, whose extensive work on the benefits of community was discussed earlier, touch on this point:

Participation and engagement result from the enactment of potential ties in real life activity. Getting together with friends, attending social functions, participating in occupational or social roles, group recreation, church attendance— these are all instances of social engagement. Thus, through opportunities for engagement, social networks define and reinforce meaningful social roles including parental, familial, occupational, and community roles, which in turn, provides a sense of value, belonging, and attachment. Those roles that provide each individual with a coherent and consistent sense of identity are only possible because of the network context which provides the theatre in which role performance takes place. In addition, network participation provides opportunities for companionship and sociability. We ... argue that these behaviors and attitudes are not the result of the provision of support per se, but are the consequence of participation in a meaningful social context in and of itself. We hypothesize that part of the reason measures of social integration or "connectedness" have been such powerful predictors of mortality for long periods of follow-up is that these ties give meaning to an individual's life by virtue of enabling him or her to participate in it fully, to be obligated (in fact, often to be the provider of support) and to feel attached to one's community.[23]

During the months following my return from Patagonia, I settled back into mainstream life, enjoying the running water, climate control, and creature comforts of my city apartment. I still felt connected to the larger community of wilderness adventurers out there in the world, shopping at the Patagonia store with increased confidence, talking crampons and kayak maneuvers with the best of them. By day I explored graduate school options and by night I organized my wilderness scrapbook, thinking about my next big adventure. Soon I was off to the suburbs of Chicago where I would study at Northwestern University and earn a master's degree in learning disabilities. This reentry into academia would be the beginning of many years of post-graduate schooling. And this next chapter in my life would involve yet another powerful experience of community, this time based on intellectual pursuits.

It Hit Me Like a Ton of Bricks

Returning to San Francisco from Chicago with my new master's degree, I resumed my running routines with varied and creative routes. The famed hills of the landscape can turn any run into an intense incline workout. One of the flattest, most beautiful and popular runs in the city is the stretch along Crissy Field, at the base of the Golden Gate Bridge. Back in the 1990s I was a regular on this route, taking in the ocean air and the view of the Bay as I got my heart pumping. On one particular day in March of 1998, I was listening to my walkman while running on the path dedicated to bikers and pedestrians that lined the road. The day was crystal clear, with blue skies and a slight breeze—the kind of day that makes you run a little faster and feel happy to be alive. The next thing I knew, I was hit by a car from behind, propelled many feet in the air, crashing to the asphalt on my right side. Dazed, confused, and unable to get up, I focused on the gashes and abrasions on my bloodied face. I remember people running over, saying things like, "She's lucky to be alive!" and "How did that happen?" When the paramedics arrived, one of them told me that I must have an angel looking out for me. I kept asking about my face and how bad the damage was; it felt like the right side of my face was barely intact. The paramedics were more concerned about my bones and the likelihood of internal injuries.

During the ugly phase of reading witness accounts and gathering information for insurance reports, I would find out that numerous bystanders had tried to flag down the driver, yelling and gesturing that she had veered off the road and was driving on the running path, but to no avail. I would also learn that the woman who hit me was ninety-one years old and that she was taking a number of medications that can affect one's driving skills. During my rehab after the accident, TJ and I saw the movie, *As Good as It Gets*, starring Jack Nicholson and Helen Hunt. It was a drama—the story of an obsessive-compulsive man and his desire for relationships. It was filled with psychological and emotional content of the kind that can make you leave the theater deep in thought about your own relationships and psychological standing. As we walked out of the theater, holding back tears, still wounded from the accident, I told TJ that I wanted to become a psychologist.

A few months after my encounter with *As Good as It Gets*, I matriculated at the Wright Institute, a clinical psychology doctoral program in Berkeley. On the second day of school, I went to my student mailbox and grabbed the stack of brochures, flyers, and other new student information inside. The first brochure I saw was an announcement for a lecture series named for a woman who had contributed much to the field of psychoanalysis in California. Her name was unique and startlingly familiar. There was no way there could be two of the same. The woman whose name was attached to the lecture series announced on this flyer in my mailbox was the same woman who had run me over at Crissy Field six months earlier.

There are moments in life when you have the feeling that things are happening for a reason, that divine intervention is at hand, or there is some grand plan for the universe. I'm not often inclined to think this way, but as I stood there staring at that flyer—my heart thumping, palms sweating, and legs shaking—I became a believer. Call it corny, mystical, what have you. The sense I made of that freakish coincidence was that I had clearly landed in the right place and was meant to study psychology. That was as good an explanation as I could come up with at the time, and to this day I haven't come up with anything better.

As it turns out, I *had* landed in the right place and proceeded to make use of the resources available to me en route to becoming a Doctor of Psychology. The combination of coursework and clinic requirements in a clinical psychology program can be intense, but I was fascinated by both aspects of the program. Classes were small and students got to know each other quite well, especially as our personalities and individual psychologies interacted with class content and with our clinic work. My favorite part of the program was the case conference where we would present case material and discuss how we were treating our clients and the reasoning behind our decisions. These seminars were the real deal—forcing us to reckon with our own experiences, emotions, defenses, and blind spots, all within a group dynamic which became part of the learning process. Once again, I had placed myself in a setting in which human nature and relational factors comprised the core of the experience. This time, my academic and clinical skills were sharpened, thanks to a community of learners and instructors who were willing to make themselves vulnerable, opening their psyches to each other and to the material with which we all grappled.

We were a community of learners engaged in the shared task of developing a greater understanding of the human experience. The community component allowed for the kind of support necessary to endure the four to six years of clinical psychology training. Our community would extend from classmates and professors to supervisors in the field and the larger network of psychologists and professors in the Bay Area. Studies have shown that learning communities can have positive benefits on student outcomes. In their two-year longitudinal study of college students, Waldron and Yungbluth looked at the effects of learning communities on participants' GPA, retention, and credit completion. They found that an increase in communication between students and faculty, with heightened experiences of social integration and opportunities for student support, all led to significant improvements in student outcomes.[24]

Much as physical vulnerability can lead to increased needs for community and social support, psychological vulnerability does so as well. To say that the process of becoming a psychologist involves emotional vulnerability might be the understatement of the year, and the need for community is paramount. I was fortunate to have been surrounded by a supportive community during my years of study, and I would argue that if, as a culture, we were to build structured communities of learners within academic fields, we would see significant positive results in our colleges and universities across all disciplines.

A poignant expression of the importance of community to the learning process comes from William J. Bauer. Writing about his experience as a Native American student advancing through the ranks of higher education, Bauer reminds his fellow Native American students, and all of us in the process, to accept the support of community and allow it to do for them as it did for him:

> *As far as advice for current and future Native scholars, I offer this: Remember your community. Given the dearth of American Indians in academia, it is safe to say that Native communities cannot always boast of their own academics. It is important to remember, however, that because of our rarity we have community and family members on reservations or in other Indian communities who overtly and tacitly support us. They provide strength when times get tough and a haven in which to recuperate.*[25]

Finding CrossFit—Community Redefined

The beginning of my career as a psychologist coincided with the beginning of my life as a mother. Earlier, I mentioned some of the challenges I faced as a new parent and some of the cultural influences at work in the experience of isolation shared by many new moms. One of the ways in which I maintained connections with other adults during those early baby-rearing years while on maternity leave from work was to spend time at our gym, then called Personal Fitness of Marin. In addition to these encounters, the most significant community experience in our lives at this time was provided by the extension of the mom's group I had joined. We would gather at each other's homes for birthday parties and other social events, husbands, babies, and toddlers in tow. This provided a sense of comfort and social connectedness with other families going through what TJ and I had come to call "The Bull's-eye Years," referring to that challenging, critical time when your children are most dependent and at their neediest. There is no respite from parenting, especially during those nights when you crave uninterrupted sleep. For us, the Bull's-eye Years were when our daughters were between the ages of one and four.

When we emerged from those early, hazy years, I was back at work doing assessments of teenagers who were acting out or struggling with learning difficulties that proved perplexing and challenging to their teachers and parents. I loved my work but it was also incredibly stressful and emotionally taxing. My schedule was tight: I was up early with the girls each workday morning and would feed and dress them, still half asleep, in order to get them off to preschool on time, before commuting to San Francisco. I would check my clothes for remnants of milk or other evidence of my children, a ritual I'm sure I shared with most working moms of toddlers and babies. This was an attempt to recapture some bit of lost dignity while also maintaining a professional standard. It was often a losing battle.

Still, life was full and rich and good, despite the hectic schedule and constant fatigue. I managed to maintain an exercise routine that helped sustain my sanity as I struggled to reclaim my pre-baby body. What I thought possible at the time was nothing like the expanded notion of the possible I know now, with CrossFit in my life. Our perceptions of what is possible in life are often vastly different from reality. My wilderness instructors used to hammer home this idea that perceived risk is very different from actual risk, whether with regard to our bodies or our minds. For me, coming from a risk-averse family culture, perceived risk was usually greater than actual risk. Perceived possibilities work in a similar way and, given my upbringing, what I thought could be possible was often limited and constrained.

There was nothing really missing from our lives during those early years with our girls. Sure, we weren't able to pay all our bills and were borrowing money from my parents, but we didn't yearn for something we didn't have. We had friends, jobs, healthy children, a house in the suburbs, and two cars to navigate it all. What I have since come to understand is that you may not know what has been missing until you discover it, and you can't imagine the possibilities until they begin to unfold.

When TJ found CrossFit and started incorporating it into his personal fitness goals and with his clientele at the gym, we had no way of knowing how it would expand and grow. The community that would develop through the vehicle of TJ's Gym/CrossFit has proven to be a real human force, powerful and inspiring. Together, we have shed pounds, raised money for those in need, helped each other through difficult times, welcomed babies, and become fitter by the day. Our lives have changed for the better and we will forever be open to the potential of a group of people sharing a passion for something positive. We will never doubt the power of a pat on the back or an encouraging cheer or a note expressing praise. We will always be aware that people can, and usually do, perform better in groups and that our potential is limited mostly by how we think about the possibilities and what we tell ourselves about our limitations.

During my research on the importance of communities, I came across a number of powerful expressions about what can happen when people come together with a common goal or shared passion. I found this comment by Polish sociologist, Zygmunt Bauman, to be particularly moving:

[I]n a community we can count on each other's good will. If we stumble and fall, others will help us to stand on our feet again. No one will poke fun at us, no one will ridicule our clumsiness and rejoice in our misfortune. If we do take a wrong step, we can still confess, explain, and apologize, repent if necessary; people will listen with sympathy and forgive us so that no one will hold a grudge forever. And there will always be someone to hold our hand at moments of sadness. When we fall on hard times and we are genuinely in need, people won't ask us for collateral before deciding to bail us out of trouble; they won't be asking us how and when will we repay, but what our needs are. And they will hardly ever say that helping us is not their duty and refuse to help us because there is no contract between us obliging them to do so, or because we failed to read the small print of the contract properly. Our duty, purely and simply, is to help each other, and so our right, purely and simply, is to expect that the help we need will be forthcoming.[26]

Great things can happen within the boundaries of a nurturing group and a collective spirit. In CrossFit the heart of connection is the willingness to push through perceived physical and psychological limitations. It is the ability to become comfortable with the uncomfortable. It is the desire to better oneself, through improved physical fitness and the awareness that doing so requires repeated and ongoing effort. It is realizing that reliance on others for support and guidance is essential, as is accepting that others are also relying on you. It means letting people of all walks of life come into yours and being open to the possibility that every one of them might be helpful to you in some way.

Despite its reputation in some circles for being a hard-core exercise program, appropriate only for the young and fit and elite athletes among us, CrossFit is actually accessible to people of all ages and fitness levels. All are welcome and each newcomer is encouraged to give it a try, at appropriate levels and with appropriate modifications. The idea is that everyone can make changes for the better, so long as they are willing to work hard and persevere in the face of challenges. As I have explained to my mother countless times over the past three years, there truly is a place for anyone within the community of CrossFit, but that does not mean that CrossFit is for everyone. A certain level of commitment is required in order to stick with a program that challenges beyond one's comfort zone. One must also have a desire and drive to work through the physical challenges set in one's path, and one must be willing to be vulnerable during the process. For those ready to commit with motivation and an openness to learn and to take on new challenges and have fun along the way, there is a place within the CrossFit community.

Margie's Story

Margie first came to TJ for personal training during her pregnancy with her second child. Having remained relatively fit during pregnancy number one, Margie was determined to do even better the second time around, despite her busy schedule as a full-time working mom with a baby at home. Her job required frequent travel, which made sticking with an exercise routine that much more challenging, but Margie was committed. After about a year of training this way and during her second postpartum struggle to regain her body, she continued to work out with TJ as he discovered CrossFit and began introducing some of its movements and methodologies to Margie and other athletes at the gym. Margie would see the people filtering into the gym for classes after her private sessions with TJ. Initially, Margie declined TJ's offers for her to join the groups; she felt the whole group exercise thing wasn't her style and she didn't think her personality was suited to the group workout experience. Gradually, Margie began to notice how much fun the class attendees seemed to be having in their group sessions. She starting getting to know some of them through conversations at the gym and gradually became interested in giving the classes a try. In early 2008, Margie bit the bullet and joined TJ's CrossFit classes with an unlimited, long-term membership.

Soon after becoming a class regular, Margie recognized the benefits of CrossFit and the group experience:

The level of intensity far surpassed anything I've experienced elsewhere in terms of the constant challenge of myself, opportunity to grow stronger, and feeling a sense of accomplishment. An enormous part of the experience is the sense of community—the connection to people that is forged through sharing intense physical and emotional experiences.

Still, Margie understood that it often takes time for her to develop close friendships, and her relationships with her classmates did not deepen right away. While she was chatty with people during warm-ups and cool downs, her interactions with her gym buddies did not extend beyond gym hours. She did feel close to TJ, however, having worked out with him for as long as she had. Margie recalls that she loved the energy of TJ's six AM group and thought that deeper connections might develop over time, but she had no idea how much this group would come to mean to her.

On August 24, 2008, approximately six months after Margie began taking group classes at TJ's Gym, her thirty-two-year-old brother fell two stories out of an apartment building in New York City, sustaining a traumatic brain injury and severe physical injuries. Margie's parents were visiting her in Marin when her father received the call all parents dread. Margie and her parents arranged to fly to New York on the red-eye that same night. This was one of those life-changing moments she will never forget:

Sitting on the airplane at 10 PM that night, the enormity of what had happened hit me, and I was terrified. With my family at home in Marin, and my parents in another part of the plane, I felt entirely alone and unprepared for what was ahead. I was doing my best to think positive thoughts about Joe, but I felt so small and insubstantial—that there was nothing I could do on my own to help Joe. I am an extremely practical person who finds it hard to stomach anything remotely resembling touchy-feely new age beliefs. But dire circumstances can cause you to depart from the norm. Sitting on the runway at Oakland, it occurred to me that a large collection of people thinking about Joe could just possibly make a difference. And I knew exactly who could make that happen. I turned on my phone and texted TJ, telling him what had happened, and asking him to ask the gym to send all their positive thoughts to my brother.

Seeing Joe for the first time after his accident was as traumatic as you would expect. He was in a coma, wrapped in bandages from head to toe, and he was hooked up to a dozen different machines, most of which were beeping. It was surreal—watching my younger brother fighting for his life, my family in shock, Joe's flood of friends crowding the waiting room—there was nothing about this experience that I knew how to handle.

TJ had emailed me and called me immediately from California, to check in on me and to see how Joe was doing. What I learned

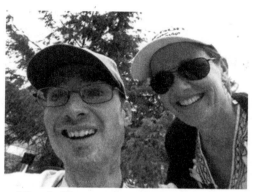

Margie Simenstad and her brother, Joe.

later in the day, when I had a chance to look at my computer, was that upon receiving my text, TJ had immediately posted something on the blog about my brother, asking for everyone's support. That's when TJ's community stepped up. A flood of emails and phone calls hit—people offering support, good thoughts, help with my kids, and kind words. People I knew casually and not at all sent the most caring and concerned messages to me—I was buoyed by the support at a time when I most needed a lift. The messages kept coming the entire week, and I know that those words of support, and the idea that so many people at home were holding Joe in their thoughts, kept me going through some very dark moments. Within a couple of days of the accident, TJ posted a WOD [Workout of the Day] called "Margie" and asked everyone to do it thinking of my brother and my family. I was so moved by this, and that week I realized quite clearly and profoundly how lucky I was to have joined the community at TJ's Gym.

Over the weeks and months that followed, Margie returned to New York regularly, making the cross-country trek and leaving behind her husband and children. The demands of this travel and care-giving schedule were extreme, but Margie didn't see it as a choice; it was simply something she and her family had to do. Now more than three years after the accident, Margie's brother has made significant progress, but he is not the same person he was before. Formerly an avid runner, he can no longer walk, and he has lost the use of his left arm. While his cognition is intact and his general mental ability has returned, his speech is impaired and he has some memory loss. Once a stand-up comedian on the New York circuit, Joe is now compromised in areas that previously made him unique. Aware enough to recognize his limitations, Joe continues his fight, with the help of Margie and other devoted family members.

During the past two years, Margie has navigated her time at the gym, diligently tracking her workouts and making great strides in areas she never thought possible—who could have imagined that she would care about her max clean and jerk? (A clean and jerk is an Olympic weightlifting movement). She has fought injuries and suffered minor setbacks, she has been derailed by work, travel and her kids' stomach bugs, but through it all Margie has persevered. She is a CrossFitter through and through and feels a deep connection to the community that has been her home in both good and challenging times. More importantly, Margie's experiences since her brother's accident have given her great insight into herself and those around her:

In addition to gratitude for the friendships I have developed, I have a new appreciation for my ability to push my body every day in the ways that CrossFit demands. ... Every day that I am in the gym, I think of Joe—I think of the things that I can do, that are painful, that are hard, that frustrate me, and I think how Joe can't even try to do them, and may never do those things again, and I am grateful for all of the challenges and the fact that I can be there to take them on. Every day, just being able to stand up and move without assistance is a gift—Joe has taught me that lesson, and my gym gives me the opportunity to appreciate it.

Margie's reflections on the role of TJ's Gym community are poignant and meaningful. Clearly, there is something powerful that continues to flourish within these walls and it is people like Margie who sustain it and give it life. Indeed, it was Margie who subsequently spearheaded a meal rotation when one of our members was diagnosed with breast cancer. This is not just a gym or lifestyle change; in Margie's own words:

> *I am not overstating things when I say that the support I got from the TJ's community during the time around Joe's accident changed my life. A group of people that I perceived as casual acquaintances stepped up and provided support that I will never forget.*

When my first draft of Margie's story was completed, it ended here. Life throws us curveballs, though, and within three months of my publication deadline, Margie received news that would change her story, and her life, and I am compelled to include an update.

Margie was diagnosed with breast cancer in the summer of 2011, at the age of forty-six. She found a lump in her breast just days after her dog had died of cancer, and it took her some time to summon the courage to make an appointment for a biopsy. Margie's Ob-Gyn gave her the unfortunate results by phone, and Margie immediately needed to visit with a primary care physician to get the full report. It was 5:00 PM on a Monday, and Margie panicked as she tried to find child care for her daughters so that she and her husband could drive to the doctor's office. After about twenty-five phone calls and twenty-five voice messages, Margie got through to a good friend—one of the coaches at TJ's Gym—who babysat while coaching an evening class. Understandably, Margie recalls being completely taken aback by the news of her cancer when it first hit:

I felt shocked, and the diagnosis was so surreal I couldn't even feel scared at first. As far as I knew I had no breast cancer in my family, I am healthy, young—this was the last thing that I thought would happen to me. Cancer has always seemed like the worst possible thing that could happen to someone— years of watching TV movies about people getting cancer, and hearing horror stories has given it a reputation probably far worse than it deserves.

Almost immediately, she and her husband went into research mode; Margie works in the health care field so she knew where to start. Her husband is a teacher who tends to gather all available data prior to making decisions. A treatment plan for cancer raises the stakes, and Margie and Chris became investigators extraordinaires, leaving no leaf unturned in their search for the best course for treatment for Triple-Negative—the aggressive form of cancer Margie faced. "Feeling fully informed helped us feel like we could tackle this and gave us more power in the situation."

However, in these circumstances, knowledge can have a downside as well. Finding out about the severity of one's illness, especially when there is a not-so-promising prognosis, can be daunting at best and paralyzing at worst. Margie recalls:

About a week after my diagnosis, I was researching Triple-Negative online and had the realization that I could die from this cancer. I felt terrified for my family—I did not want my girls to lose their mother, Chris to lose his wife. That was the one day that I felt scared. After that, I chose to think only positively and have felt very optimistic since.

Margie has followed a path of optimism and strength so far. Although she admits to being tired from her chemotherapy treatments from time to time, she is taking on this battle in the best way she knows how—armed with positive thinking, reliance on friends and well-wishers, and with a dogged determination to beat the disease so that she can be around for her girls as they grow up.

Margie is not alone in this fight, a fact that comforts her in her toughest moments. She knows from firsthand experience with her brother's accident and subsequent medical challenges that the power of a group of supporters is essential to psychological survival when the going gets extra tough. Margie has, once again, benefited from the army of friends and acquaintances she has made in her four years at TJ's Gym. Leading the charge has been one of Margie's coaches and close friends, Toni, who has, among other things, distributed Team Margie bracelets to the entire gym population, organized a hike to raise money for breast cancer in Margie's honor, and raised funds for a housekeeping service to help Margie with household chores.

> *Something changed for me a couple of weeks in—maybe it was ... the Team Margie bracelets. Seeing my friends, and even people I didn't know very well, wearing the bracelets has such a positive effect on my spirit and attitude and it has been amazing to see people wearing them. I actually saw someone I didn't know wearing one at a stoplight once. So many people from TJ's have sent me notes and talked to me at the gym, sharing their support, and even their own experiences with cancer. ... My TJ's community is actually a lot bigger than I thought. It's not just the 5:15 crew, but the people that come in for the 6:15 class, the people on the discussion board that I don't know very well, the coaches—the support and love never cease to surprise me, and mean so much to me.*

Much as she did after her brother's crisis, Margie has spent time reflecting on how it is that a group of people—a community sharing common ground—can propel an individual through grief, fear, pain, and even the fight for her life. She speaks not only of the leadership

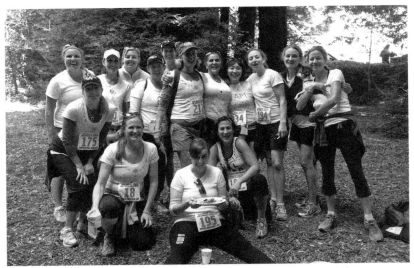

***Margie and a group of TJ's Gym supporters on a hike
for breast cancer research.***

that sets the tone for a group but also the core idea that ties together the stories in this book: connections grounded and created in a shared physical struggle are connections that have a special meaning and power.

> *I don't know exactly what the secret ingredient is of TJ's. Part of it is TJ—he is so compassionate and cares deeply about everyone, and we all have taken on that quality too, or feel more free to share it with each other. Another part is that bonds are forged that are rooted in strength and determination. These are prized qualities at TJ's, and we all see them in each other, and encourage each other to bring them out. At first we view these from a purely physical perspective, but as we get to know each other, we all bring our best to the table to support each other, no matter what we are facing.*

Margie is bound and determined to triumph over her latest life challenge. She will again face the future with her incredible spirit and positive attitude, combined with the support of almost 1,000 TJ's members and friends behind her. Her sister's recent diagnosis of breast cancer has increased the trauma for this family. But they are strong and courageous and they will fight. And the community will be there for them.

Chapter 6

Are Communities Always Positive Forces?

So far, we have seen how communities can be social tools for bringing out the best in their members. We've seen how community affiliation can provide solace for people in need, can drive people to perform and learn, can push people beyond perceived limitations, and can help people deal with illness and challenging life events.

But what about the potential downside of people coming together and sharing negative or even dangerous ideas, philosophies, and goals? What about communities whose leaders have problematic or even antisocial aims and who convince others to follow them? What about communities whose members—attracted to, or even seduced by, the possibility for connection—end up doing bad things to others in order to sustain their communal ties? Even Putnam, who, as we have seen, is an enthusiastic advocate for communities and the power of social capital, acknowledges the potential for social capital to be misused in antisocial ways. Citing such examples as the Holocaust, the KKK, and Timothy McVeigh and his cohorts in the Oklahoma City bombing, Putnam explains, "Social capital, in short, can be directed toward malevolent, antisocial purposes, just like any other form of capital."[27] History is replete with stories of people who have managed to attract others to a group and use that affinity for harmful ends.

If human nature includes a drive to cultivate extra-familial ties, it comes as no surprise that social ties will develop across a variety of demographic and psychological lines. When all goes well within family relationships and when basic psychological needs are met, individuals are often motivated to connect at the next level, within a group sharing a common pursuit, mission, or philosophy. These communal networks are not meant to take the place of the family bond but rather are supplemental avenues for human connection. However, when family relationships are compromised or psychological needs go unmet, people may be left craving connections in a less grounded way. Without a positive force or role model available to steer these people towards positive social connections, these subgroups can be based on unconscious and sometimes destructive needs. Such community relationships are likely to be volatile, unpredictable, and unproductive, both for the people within them and for society at large. We might compare the example of the neglected adolescent girl whose sexual promiscuity is a misguided attempt at intimacy, to an antisocial community with its manipulative methods of seeking social capital and cohesion.

We can easily imagine the development of community support and engagement in the lives of children whose fundamental needs are met as they grow; my personal history is an example of this trajectory. However, for children whose lives are marked by a poverty of relationship and a lack of psychological stability or sense of security, social affiliation comes with complications and the potential for harm. For children and teens raised in inner cities who are exposed to violence, poverty, drug abuse, neglect, and an experience of marginalization, the likelihood that social connectedness might be possible or beneficial becomes increasingly remote. Typically, these young people are shown over and over again that others are not to be trusted and that "looking out for number one" is the only way to survive. Psychological and emotional wellness are luxuries not available to kids who are often fighting for their very lives; they are focused on physical safety and basic security, lacking role models to forge a path of relational health and social well-being. Still, the fundamental and relational needs of these kids are similar to those of their more privileged peers. All too often, the young people of our cities fall prey to gangs and malevolent groups that offer some kind of connection in an otherwise alienating world. Writing on this topic, Princeton University Sociology Professor Alejandro Portes explains:

Whereas bounded solidarity and trust provide the sources for socioeconomic ascent and entrepreneurial development among some groups, among others they have exactly the opposite effect. Sociability cuts both ways. While it can be the source of public goods ... it can also lead to public "bads." Mafia families, prostitution and gambling rings, and youth gangs offer so many examples of how embeddedness in social structures can be turned to less than socially desirable ends.[28]

Many researchers who explore the potential downside of social capital and communities gone awry note how groups of marginalized people often become dependent on negative insider status. Their connection, based on exclusion of outsiders and an experience of being cast aside, is likely to lead to negative outcomes. We see this played out again and again in urban gangs across America where the ties that bind are ties built on the experience of "us against them." It becomes critically important, then, that membership stays within.

Portes notes that "there are situations in which group solidarity is cemented by a common experience of adversity and opposition to mainstream society. ... The result is downward leveling norms that operate to keep members of a downtrodden group in place and force the more ambitious to escape from it."[29]

Zygmunt Bauman, author of *Community: Seeking Safety in an Insecure World*, describes this downward spiral:

> *Ghetto life does not sediment community. Sharing stigma and public humiliation does not make the sufferers into brothers; it feeds mutual derision, contempt, and hatred. A stigmatized person may like or dislike another bearer of stigma, stigmatized individuals may live in peace or be at war with each other— but one thing they are unlikely to do is to develop mutual respect. "The others like me" means the others unworthy as I myself have been repeatedly told that I am and been shown to be; "to be more like them" means to be more unworthy than I already am.*[30]

It is important to note that while gangs may permeate our inner cities, another form of negative community has developed in more privileged settings. An unfortunate trend among teens and young adults in suburban and mainstream America involves the severe bullying and exclusion of individuals by groups of fellow high school and college students. Internet social networks have reinforced the negative consequences of such peer pressure. Recently, stories of teen suicides in response to these behaviors have shocked a number of middle-class and upper-middle-class communities. In such cases, parents, teachers, and counselors are forced to reckon with the dangerous results of these peer groups united around making others feel unworthy and unwelcome. Perhaps this exclusion gives young people a sense of security in their own social standing. Whatever the motivations, these groups are examples of how social affinities in more privileged areas can have as insidious an impact as gangs in the inner city.

We have seen that gang membership is consistent with the human drive to connect and enjoy social affiliation, but limited by negative environmental influences. Perhaps, then, an antidote to gang membership might be the introduction and availability of affiliations using positive role models and mentors. Boys and Girls Clubs across the country have long since striven for, and achieved in large measure, this kind of forum for underprivileged youth. On a smaller scale, but growing steadily, Steve's Club is doing the same.

The Story of Steve and his Club

Steve Liberati grew up in a blue-collar neighborhood in Gloucester Township, New Jersey, located between Philadelphia and Camden, New Jersey. His father was an exterminator who ran his own business, and his mother worked in a doctor's office. Steve is the second oldest of four children—he has an older brother and two younger sisters. The family lived in a small, three-bedroom ranch house. Quarters were tight, but they managed. The Liberatis are Catholic which, to Steve, meant saying grace before dinner, attending an occasional Sunday Mass, and taking part in most of the sacraments of the Church. While he attended Catholic school from elementary through high school, Steve was somewhat skeptical of the teachings of the Church, tending to question and think for himself.

Steve was an avid athlete, playing baseball, basketball, floor hockey, and wrestling, participating on teams throughout his school years. Like many young people who join in team sports, Steve learned about relationships and navigated his social world through these experiences: "Playing on sports teams had a huge impact on my life and helped me form the person I am today. It taught me to put the team before myself and to cooperate with others, especially kids from diverse backgrounds and with different personality types. Most importantly, sports taught me that hard work was a requirement if I wanted to succeed. Like most kids, I was not given any special talents, so I had to work extra hard to improve my skills on the field."

In addition to organized sports, Steve and the other neighborhood kids had lots to do. They were fortunate to live near well-maintained baseball fields for pickup sandlot games, a lake in which to fish, and expansive backyards where they could play freely and do what kids do. Steve recalls having a strong group of friends in elementary school and high school, which provided a secure sense of belonging and acceptance: "I'm a big believer that you are who you hang out with. ... One of my favorite quotes is, 'those who lie down with dogs get up with fleas.'"

Steve learned early on the value of hard work. Although his parents were willing to provide for the needs of their children, the message that nothing in life is free was communicated early and often by Steve's hardworking father who would tell him: "everything worth having is earned." Steve worked throughout his school years— for spending money and to earn his keep—first with a newspaper route and later for his father by day and at a local GNC store at night. He continued to work through college, helping to pay his tuition and monthly expenses. While many of his friends and classmates spent their time studying and partying, Steve worked more than twenty-five hours a week with the satisfaction and conviction that "things should never come easy." At the time, he imagined that he would eventually rise through the ranks on Wall Street or become some kind of entrepreneur.

After Steve's graduation from the University of Delaware, the allure of security and a possible career path led him to accept a job at a large bank. Steve recalls, "the job sounded great and had a nice title and made my parents proud, but it was clear to me that it was something I couldn't do for a lifetime. ... I called it the corporate treadmill. I was running nowhere fast. ... I was making decent money, but I did not receive any personal reward or satisfaction from it. It was only a paycheck." In May 2007, driven to find something more fulfilling, Steve started working for his father's extermination business with the idea that he would eventually run it himself.

Many of his father's accounts were in nearby Camden, a city that consistently has one of the highest crime rates in the country. Steve worked in the housing projects there, noticing the local youth hanging out in the neighborhood streets. As he became a familiar presence, he would ask them questions about sports and working out, which provided some common ground. The boys in Camden reminded Steve of himself at their age—trying to find things to do to stay out of trouble after school. But Camden's reputation was not good: the streets were rougher than the grasses of Steve's hometown and the kids roaming the streets were reportedly more dangerous.

As it turned out, in Steve's experience, the stereotypes didn't always hold up, and he looked forward to his interactions with the kids when he traveled to Camden. He soon realized that these were "normal" kids who happened to be surrounded by gangs, violence, and drugs. It was an environment that was not conducive to a healthy or productive lifestyle, to say the least, and the temptations were pervasive and seductive. The kids Steve saw were at a crossroads— age twelve, thirteen, pre-drug use and pre-gang—but the bad stuff was there waiting for them, beckoning at every corner, with the promise of escape and empowerment.

One of Steve's passions in those days was doing something called CrossFit. He had happened upon the program through a blog he frequented, written by author Seth Godin.[31] Interested in forces of change in our society, Godin wrote about how CrossFit was sparking a revolution in fitness. Curious and intrigued, Steve was giving CrossFit a shot, doing the workouts from Crossfit.com by himself in the local gym where he was a member. Steve remembers the "rude awakening" of realizing how far he was from being truly fit. He was hooked! Steve would talk about his fitness routines with the boys of

Camden and at some point it occurred to him—and them—that they might get together for some workouts. The rest, as they say, is history.

Steve's Club was first housed in the community center of Centennial Village Apartments, a public housing complex. There, Steve trained the kids of Camden, meeting them in between working appointments for his dad's company. The group grew quickly and Steve knew he was onto something. While he had little, if any, contact with their parents, he knew he was having a positive impact on these young people. The majority of Steve's kids came from homes with single mothers, and they lacked a father figure in their lives. Steve was pleased to fill that role, even if only for brief periods each week. His own family was supportive of his efforts, with some reservations. Steve's wife was concerned about his safety and also worried about the significant time commitment. The couple did not have children of their own, but she still worried about his availability for her and the family. After all, Steve worked full days with his father and then spent two hours training the Steve's Club kids, driving them to and from the gym. In addition, he lived forty-five minutes from Camden, adding a major commute to his already stretched day. Steve's father shared his daughter-in-law's concerns at first, but eventually came around.

After about a year, Steve's Club lost its use of the Centennial Village community center, due to a scheduling conflict with another after-school program. Space was surprisingly difficult to find. Despite a plethora of run-down, vacant buildings, apparently nobody was interested in leasing to Steve. He approached schools, churches, and assorted other institutions, many of which had room to spare. He wasn't asking for money. Still, he was refused time and time again. Ultimately, after much searching, Steve secured a space borrowed from the Police Athletic League on the other side of town. Using his own savings, he bought a van to cart the kids to and from their gym, parking it in a fenced lot when not in use. Camden has the highest incidence of car theft of any city in the United States (from Steve's

Club website). And as it turns out, Camden had the highest overall crime rate of any U.S. city in 2008, with 2,333 violent crimes for every 100,000 residents, compared to the national average of 455 per 100,000.[32] Steve and his kids persisted throughout the year despite another location change, training indoors and outside at a local park, even in inclement weather.

The following comment on the Steve's Club website describes the Camden bureaucracy:

The greatest discovery any alien outsider could make about Camden is its overriding response to failure: If it didn't work last year, do it AGAIN this year (and if possible do it MORE). Every year they pass more laws, hire more police, build more prisons, and sentence more offenders for longer periods—all without moving one inch closer to "ending" crime. ... Every year they spend more money on schools, hoping to "fix" whatever's wrong with them, and every year the schools remain stubbornly unfixed. ... Every year they try to make the criminals go away, and every year they remain with us. We couldn't shoehorn these criminals back into the "the mainstream" last year or the year before that or the year before that or the year before that, but you can be sure we'll try it again this year, knowing beyond a shadow of a doubt that it won't work this year either. Maybe it's time to try something different.[33]

During the early years of Steve's Club, Steve was becoming increasingly passionate about sharing CrossFit with others in the community. As he gathered momentum with the Club, he was also training more and more adults he would meet at the park with the kids. While Steve was committed to working with the kids long term, he was also practical and knew that he needed income to keep it all going. Steve subsequently founded CrossFit Tribe, a CrossFit

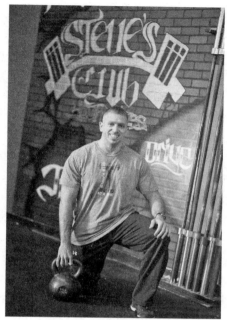

Steve Liberati

affiliate whose members could afford to pay dues. He chose the name to reflect his experience of two communities coming together and also to acknowledge the aspect of evolutionary fitness inherent in CrossFit. Steve also credits Seth Godin's book, *Tribes*, as influencing him in his choice of name. Godin writes of the human drive to form tribes and the ways in which we can become leaders and agents of change in our world.[34] Steve was inspired, and CrossFit Tribe was born.

In September 2008, CrossFit Tribe and Steve's Club opened their doors in a new shared space. According to Steve, "It was great having them next door to each other. The two communities exchanged energy and fed off each other. The members of Tribe were inspired by the kids, and the kids got to meet the adults and build relationships with them." Although the space was small and modest, these two groups were coming together as one, clearly thriving within those walls.

Over time, as Steve and his kids connected in deeper ways, Steve understood the positive impact he could have on their young lives.

In October 2008, in response to complaints from some of the most committed of Steve's Clubbers about the unhealthy food choices at the school cafeteria, Steve and his wife began making nutritious snacks and small meals for the kids to bring to school. They were sent off with beef jerky, nuts, and berries in plastic baggies—a kind of armor against the fried food and sugar of the lunch lines. In time, supported by Steve's entrepreneurial spirit, these small meals became "PaleoKits"—consistent with CrossFit's emphasis on eating a paleo diet. The diet is rooted in the kinds of foods our pre-argrarian ancestors ate—lean meats, fruits, vegetables, healthy unsaturated fats, limited sugar, and no processed foods. While the Paleo diet is chosen for nutritional purposes with the goal of optimizing athletic performance, it also brings us back to a time when people traveled in tribes and nomadic communities—yet another communal link, this time to our past. Steve started selling PaleoKits online in order to raise funds for equipment and other program needs. He even hired some of the Steve's Club kids to pack boxes and manage inventory, thus giving them a sense of industry and an income to boot.

By August 2009, CrossFit Tribe and Steve's Club had moved again, this time to a more spacious location where they are currently housed. Kids walk, ride bikes, or get a ride in the Club van—whatever it takes to get there. These are the same kids who have been described as having no drive, work ethic, or ability to commit. Steve's Club has now evolved into a national program, with a number of CrossFit affiliates around the country providing training for kids and teens in impoverished and crime-ridden neighborhoods. The goal is "to help kids realize their greatness by training to be better athletes, students, and citizens." Steve's Club earned official nonprofit status and recently partnered with the Boys and Girls Clubs of America. Steve and his partners are in the process of creating the infrastructure that will allow the national program to gain traction and expand further.

Steve is modest about his accomplishments. He acknowledges that he has kept many kids from joining gangs, but he laments the one or two who have strayed from Steve's Club and succumbed to gang pressures. He knows that the relationships these kids develop through the Club, as well as the affinity they feel with each other and with the CrossFit community as a whole, have been life changing for many. While the process is not just about the workouts, the workouts do matter. As Steve explains:

CrossFit is the perfect hook—it's a great tool. CrossFit does a great job—it's intense, it's fun, it's constantly varied. Bodybuilding wouldn't work. The kids like competing, putting numbers on the board. CrossFit is the hook that provides the opportunity to work with the kids one-on-one and start talking to them. It's a way to offer advice, to be there as a role model, an example of something different. Plus, there's the community of CrossFit, the presence online. They can look at videos and identify with other people doing the workouts. The community becomes theirs. It's super exciting. They are part of something bigger than themselves. CrossFit is something they can see themselves in and become attached to. They feel a part of it, which, for these kids is critical. It's a good alternative to a gang, which a lot of them would otherwise get involved in. After workouts at the Club, they bond and share stories and ideas, and it's a place to get away from it all.

These sentiments are echoed by Lee Knight, program director at Steve's Club. Lee has a background in management consulting and strategic marketing and is also a CrossFit competitor. She describes the power of the experience for Steve's Club kids when they realize they are part of something bigger. Thanks to CrossFit headquarters, a group from the Club attended the CrossFit Games in July 2010 and even competed in the teen event at the Games in 2011. When athletes from other CrossFit gyms around the world come to CrossFit Tribe and Steve's Club to train, the kids see how they all speak a common language and do the same workouts. They are also aware of the many fund-raisers that are held in support of their gym, including the now annual special event, "Beat the Streets."

Lee explains that the kids "get it that people out there care about them and their population, even though they don't know them. That's really important for them. We can help one kid at a time. Even if you make a difference in only one kid's life, that will eventually reach fifteen kids. The hook is CrossFit and the physical training. It gets them in the door. They don't really know that it's hard work. It's kind of masked, but there's so much more to it. There's the good nutrition, making sure they are resting well. ... We see that they spend their off time here, and this becomes their community." Lee expresses with enthusiasm how Steve's Club is making a difference:

When we ask the kids what it means to them, they are quick to say: "If I weren't here, I would be into bad things—doing drugs, in a gang." It's less about the friends and more about a safe haven and a purpose in their lives. They care about their PRs [personal records] and their Fran times [a signature CrossFit workout]. They know that they need to be here to have that happen. It's about having a family. They are really good kids, but it's easy to see how they could get sidetracked if they were just sitting around on a stoop somewhere. This gives them a purpose—it gives them enough to say "I'm not going to do that stuff."

Jose is a nineteen-year-old member of Steve's Club who has been training there for over two years. Back in high school in Camden, Jose had tried out for the basketball team as a senior but didn't make the cut. Instead of trying to improve his game, he "just gave up." Now Jose credits Steve's Club for helping him see that you sometimes

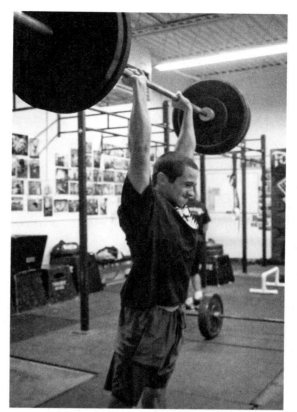

Jose, Steve's Club Member.

have to work hard in order to achieve your goals and that your goals are often worth the effort. He is currently a proud member of a church basketball team and has played in two tournaments. Jose is also pursuing school at night and has become more focused and goal-oriented in that pursuit as well.

Asked to reflect on how life at Steve's Club has affected him, Jose explains:

> *If there is one thing I took from Steve's Club into my life, it would be the motivation part, and the relationships with other people, too. I now see Steve's Club as my family. I see the*

young kids and it feels good when you can lend an open hand when they need help. ... Many times I can feel that something is needed in my life, and with God, Steve's Club, CrossFit, and my family, everything feels complete. ... My life can now easily be put in three words—focused, motivated, listener. I'm focused in one way because I stay on track with what I have to do, whether it's learning a technique in the gym or keep going to school. Motivated because I now go after the things I need without doubting myself anymore. And as a listener, I now have so much advice in my life I can write a book. Whether it was coming from my family, Steve's Club, or a stranger, I always try to listen.

For Ralf, another nineteen-year-old member of Steve's Club, CrossFitting at the club has impacted his life outside of the gym as much as his performance inside the gym. Here is his brief description of how his involvement in Steve's Club has changed his life, and how it's much more than a workout:

I have grown mentally and have learned how to stay strong, even when life throws a curve ball. Just like in a workout, I have to stay strong and keep chipping away. Steve's Club has also helped me become more social and interact with others, and it's fun knowing that I'm not as shy as before. Being in Steve's Club has actually helped me in knowing and being an example of how hard work can produce rewards. My future seems very bright and my dreams of playing college football become more and more reachable every day. ... The best parts of Steve's Club are the people, the help, and the support. It's great to know that not only can we work out, but also receive advice when something is going wrong in the rest of our life. The best part about CrossFit is the community. I know

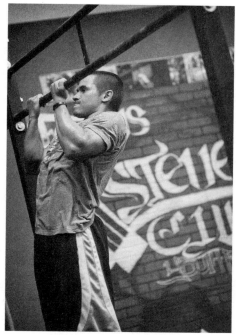

Ralf, Steve's Club Member.

deep down in my heart and soul that Steve's Club has been a blessing to me and my life.

One of the unique aspects of Steve's Club is how it acts as a tribe, a movement and following started by a dedicated and charismatic leader. As Seth Godin explains, "Tribes are about faith—about belief in an idea and in a community. And they are grounded in respect and admiration for the leader of the tribe and for the other members as well."[35] Steve's Club is a thriving, inspiring example of how commitment to a cause and the connection to a community can change people's lives.

Olivia's Story

Ah, to be sixteen in the summertime and living in the suburbs of San Francisco. Life is good around here, the weather is always sunny, and opportunities to enjoy the Great Outdoors abound. For many high schoolers in Marin County, summer is a time for jobs at camps and staying in shape for fall sports.

In the summer of 2010, Olivia was sixteen, heading into her junior year in high school, weighed 227 pounds, and had a body fat percentage of well over thirty. She was literally trapped in her body and was extremely unhealthy and inactive. Despite her size and lack of fitness, Olivia was a member of the Redwood High School cheerleading program. Her coach had connected with TJ and knew about our TEAM program (Training Elite Athletes in Marin). When she first heard of the workouts at TJ's Gym, Olivia was afraid. She heard people say things like, "that was the hardest workout I've ever done." Olivia knew she was dreadfully out of shape, but at a friend's urging, she decided to give it a try.

After her first workout, Olivia had a sense that the program could help her:

It was definitely one of the hardest things I have ever done, but for some reason I was hooked after the first workout and started coming three days a week. I don't know why I continued, and it would have been so easy for me to just quit. There was something about the way I was treated when I was there that made me feel so welcome that first time, like I could do so much more than I thought. ... For the first month, I was intimidated and scared, but the TJ's community instantly made me feel right at home. I was so surprised when people I had never met before cheered for me in a workout. That was what captured my heart. ... Once I started to see how good I felt after each workout, I began to really give each workout my all.

I loved doing CrossFit from the first workout, even though it was hard, because of the people I met at the gym. The hardest part for me in the beginning was my own insecurity. I was so self-conscious about my fitness level in the beginning. Everyone at the gym was in such good shape, and I just wanted to be able to do the things that they could.

After listening to one of TJ's nutrition talks following a TEAM class in July, Olivia went home intrigued and eager to learn more about the Paleo way of eating. She immersed herself in her research and, with her mother's approval and the encouragement of a doctor who had been concerned about her health, Olivia jumped right in. Her body responded right away. She recalls feeling dramatic changes in her energy levels, her moods, and her ability to perform during workouts. She remembers feeling "happier" just knowing that she was finally doing something good for her body and improving her lifestyle. Olivia observes:

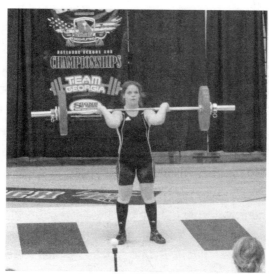

Olivia Smith competing at the Schoolage National Weightlifting Championships in Flowery Branch, Georgia. June, 2011.

The results came extremely fast. I started to lose weight within two weeks. ... After I had been in the program for a month and a half, I had lost almost twenty pounds. The speed at which my body dropped the weight is incredible. I think that shows how unhealthy I really was. My body was ready to lose as much weight as it could at the first chance it got. My family noticed the difference in me almost immediately. Then the people at the gym started to compliment the way I looked and how fit I was getting. Family members I haven't seen in a while still notice the changes. A few days ago I went to the dentist. I hadn't been in six months, and I was really surprised when the receptionist told me how great I looked. I guess when you are the one changing every day you don't notice how drastic the changes are. I still get so many people who comment on my body, which encourages me to keep losing weight. Before losing weight, I hated any attention, because I always felt like it was negative. Now I love it.

While Olivia's outward appearance has changed dramatically, what is even more powerful are the changes that have occurred within. Olivia is undeniably more self-assured, confident, happy, and optimistic than she was before coming to TJ's. She has a newfound sense of herself as a competent person whose voice should be heard, and she is more likely to assert herself in conversations. Always a great student, Olivia continues to excel in school and is now more likely to participate in activities where she once shied away. She is effervescent when reflecting on these changes within, and when she talks about them, you cannot help but share her enthusiasm.

So many people tell me how much happier I seem now. Coworkers, family members, and friends all comment on how I smile so much more and how my attitude toward life has become more positive. I also think that the confidence that I gained has improved my relationships. I stand up to people and voice my opinions more. The most important part of my success has been the community. All of the amazing people I've met who've inspired me are what keep me coming back again and again. I love everyone at the gym, the way they push each other, keep each other honest, and support each other. That's what I come back for every day. I never would have stuck it out through all the hard workouts, failed PR (Personal Record) attempts, and difficult days if it wasn't for the community. The community inspires me, and I couldn't do this without them.

Olivia's transformation is a success story in its own right but there's more: During Olivia's first TEAM session, TJ noticed that she was incredibly strong. She was able to lift weights with ease that many of our adult men can't move. She was clearly an incredibly powerful athlete, and TJ encouraged Olivia to try the Olympic Weightlifting program at our San Rafael location. Somewhat nervous at first, but with her newfound confidence and faith in the gym community behind her, Olivia began specializing in Olympic lifting. Turns out, she's not just good at it—she's gifted and great! Within months of doing her first clean and jerk, Olivia qualified for the Junior Nationals school-aged division. One of Olivia's many fans in the TJ's community took Olivia under her wing and together they solicited donations from local businesses for a raffle to raise money for Olivia to travel to Georgia for the competition. While Olivia's first national meet did not go as well as she had hoped, she is undeterred in her motivation for success in the sport and continues her training daily. Olivia has already given back to the community that has given her so much joy. She has been an assistant coach in the TJ's Kids CrossFit program, and she inspires other gym members every day with her own story and workout posts.

Olivia's future is bright. She is physically strong and healthy, and she has gained a level of self-confidence and insight rare for most seventeen-year-olds. She is no longer introverted and afraid as she navigates the world. It is difficult to capture Olivia's enthusiasm and remarkable zest for life through paraphrase; her own words tell the story best:

> *The biggest benefit for me has been how happy I have become. I am loving life. I have a second family at the gym. I am competing in a sport I love. I am surrounded by amazing people. I am healthy, and I have so much more confidence. I can't even imagine what my life would be like if I had not found TJ's and CrossFit. I would definitely not be as happy as I am now.*

One of Olivia's extracurricular activities at school is writing for the school newspaper. *The Redwood Bark* is a respected school publication whose reporters have proven to be top-notch communicators. In December 2010, Olivia wrote an Opinion article for the paper about her transformative experience at TJ's Gym. It is reproduced here in its entirety:

WORKING OUT TOGETHER LIGHTENS THE LOAD
by Olivia Smith

Squats. Double unders. Sprints. Burpees. Five months ago I would have dreaded the thought of exercising for more than ten minutes. Now my heart races with excitement at the thought of back squatting to find a new one rep max, or performing the workout of the day.

I personally struggle with my fitness and have struggled with it for my whole life. Over the last five months I have lost 65 pounds by dramatically changing my diet and exercise routine. Before losing weight, I was unhappy every day. I hated who I was because of the weight. I was introduced to a community where I found a certain kind of happiness that I had never experienced before. It was a support system that made me feel great about myself no matter how hard my day had been, how slow I performed a workout, or how out of shape I was.

In joining TJ's Gym, I replaced my unhealthy lifestyle with a new family who helped me over the peak of my weight struggle and to create a healthy lifestyle. In addition to losing weight, I found a love for a new sport. Olympic weightlifting gives me a sense of accomplishment, whether I am making a new personal record in the gym or competing for the first time in a meet. Training with the Olympic weightlifting team is the highlight of my week because my teammates make me feel great about the work that I do, no matter if I made all of my lifts or none of them.

After only a month and a half of training, I competed in my first weightlifting meet. When my nerves finally subsided, I only missed one out of my six attempts to complete lifts at increasing weights. There is not a day I can remember when I dreaded going to workout. It was not the painful workouts that have captured my heart, but the person suffering next to me, who still managed to say words of encouragement between gasps for breath. The community has a way of making a person feel important, which has the ability to save a life. The most important thing to me throughout this process was the community's ability to help me achieve success.

I went from being a cheerleader who was seventy-five pounds overweight to winning second place for my weight class in an Olympic weightlifting competition. My life is completely different, and I am finally pursuing things that make me feel great about who I am. Before I lost weight, I didn't pay much attention to what I was eating or what I was doing to take care of my body. I never realized before the importance of maintaining personal fitness in everyday life. One of the factors that can lead to happiness with who you are is being content with your own personal fitness.

Being fit is an empowering way to live life. I have seen the confidence that I gained in my body transfer into other parts of my life. I am more outgoing around my friends and willing to meet new people. I voice my opinions more and do a better job of defending them. Now I am training in the sport of Olympic weightlifting. The possibilities for the future are infinite and there is no limit to where weightlifting will take me. [36]

Chapter 7

A Community Outdoors

You've heard my personal account of my experiences with community in the backcountry of the Eastern Sierras and the wilderness of Patagonia. Many of you may have an adventuresome spirit of your own and perhaps have conquered mountain peaks, skied in remote mountain ranges, or navigated the white waters of a river. You may have encountered the sense of community shared among those involved, whether as part of a defined group venturing out together or experiencing the outdoors as individuals and crossing paths with others along the way.

When people go forth on an adventure in nature, magical things can happen. Stripped of the usual trappings of our social worlds and forced to reckon with ourselves without the luxuries of home, we tend to shift into a heightened focus on the challenges at hand, while opening ourselves to others. This might be our psychological survival mechanism kicking in—we know that if something were to go wrong in a place where our cell phones would do us no good, other people would be our only hope. Strangers heading along the same wilderness trail might just become saviors, and somewhere in the recesses of our psyches, that registers loudly and clearly.

That wilderness experiences can change people's lives and create new pathways for relationships is a concept that has been adopted extensively in the therapeutic world. Wilderness therapy programs, for example, abound for troubled adolescents. As is true of all forms of therapy, there are varying theoretical approaches and treatment philosophies, and the suitability of any one program for any one individual is multifaceted. Still, there is clearly something important and universal about the outdoor aspect of these treatments, and the group and communal elements are significant factors in creating change.

Judging from the quantity of publications and films on the subject, we are fascinated by stories of survival in the wilderness. We are captivated by the idea of testing ourselves in nature, yet we are terrified by the potential risks involved. Most of us live vicariously through media portrayals of adventurers living in the extreme, overcoming elements of nature—weather, animals, terrain, injury—ultimately emerging to tell the tale. Some of us have had a small taste of wilderness survival, while others live life on the edge all the time, perhaps driven by some unspoken force within to seek out the thrill of adventure and the rush of overcoming the odds. In my mind, there is a great crevasse (pun intended) between the psychology of soloists and those who venture out in groups. There is something dramatically different about what happens to people who are truly alone in nature and those who share the experience with others. My focus here is on the community element of outdoor adventures and what the experience of being out in a group can do for human relationships and the formation of connections.

Outdoor adventure always involves a physical component, regardless of the mode of transportation or the kind of terrain. When we are out in nature without access to running water, ready sources of food, fire, climate control, and other amenities of modern life, we must be self-reliant in order to make it through. While we don't necessarily need to be extremely fit to survive in the woods, many aspects of fitness give us obvious advantages when we are faced with the challenges of putting up a tent, hiking a steep trail, navigating rough waters, building fires, and even outrunning potential predators. It's no coincidence, then, that many outdoor adventurers prioritize their fitness training when they are between trips. Increasingly, and also not surprisingly, many are turning to CrossFit. In addition to the physical advantages CrossFit training can provide, we know that the community experience and camaraderie are also important benefits of the program. And for many outdoor adventurers accustomed to this kind of connection, the community aspect of CrossFit is a significant draw.

Brad and First Descents:
There's Something in the Waters

Throughout my research on communities and CrossFit and what fuels people to take on certain activities and make life-changing connections along the way, I was fortunate to be hooked up with a number of individuals who have created communities of their own, via their passion for a special activity and cause. It turns out that if you dig a little, you find that there are lots of amazing and inspiring stories to be told. A large part of the CrossFit ethos involves altruism and philanthropy—giving back to the larger community or taking care of people within who need help.

In CrossFit gyms worldwide, on any given weekend, there are assorted fund-raisers in action—workouts for populations in need, workouts to honor fallen heroes and raise funds for their families, workouts to raise money to fight illnesses. It's probably not a coincidence that CrossFit tends to attract people with an unusually strong sense of community and a desire to give back to others. When you combine this altruistic spirit with a love of the great outdoors and an appreciation for how wilderness experience can change lives, you can create something powerful. This is exactly what CrossFitter Brad Ludden did when he was just eighteen years old.

Since the age of thirteen, Brad has been a professional white-water kayaker. Raised in Montana, his father is a physician who worked hard to create and sustain his private practice, instilling in Brad and his sister a tenacious work ethic. Brad's mother, who had studied special education, spent her days volunteering to help populations in need. Weekends for the Ludden family were dedicated to outdoor activities: skiing, hiking, camping, kayaking, fishing, hunting, and in general, spending time together enjoying nature. According to Brad, "it was this encouragement to find peace and challenge in the outdoors that led to my special focus on kayaking."

When he was nine years old, Brad's parents bought him and his sister their first kayaks, a gift that turned out to be the beginning of a lifelong passion. When he was twelve, Brad traveled to Chile to attend a kayaking school, and when he was thirteen his parents sent him off to Colorado for a "rite of passage" experience in the outdoors. "Upon returning, they told me that I was my own person, an adult responsible for my own decisions and the consequences of those decisions. They gave me the freedom to fly and it changed my life for good." Brad first became a sponsored kayaker at age thirteen, earning significant income by the time he was seventeen. Good thing, too, because his father strongly believed that children should provide for themselves, and Brad and his sister were expected to contribute.

Brad's adolescence was different in many ways from the typical day-to-day life of an upper-middle-class kid in America. He traveled extensively throughout the world to compete in kayaking events, gaining insight into the possibilities of his privileged life. When Brad was sixteen, his aunt was diagnosed with cancer. He remembers the moment when "cancer went from being a word to being personal." Driven to do something to help, he became a volunteer in a pediatric oncology ward at a local hospital. During his time there, Brad decided he could be doing more for people with cancer: He imagined that he could take them out for kayaking trips where they would be able to get away, if only briefly, from their daily struggles with the disease.

Young people often have lofty ideals of changing the world, but few are able to make things happen. Brad was a unique case, so committed, in fact, that he decided he was ready to graduate from high school in three years to develop a nonprofit organization dedicated to guiding cancer patients on kayak excursions. When his public high school would not allow this, Brad enrolled in a kayak academy, hoping they would. When administrators there also refused early graduation, Brad persisted, finding a community college where he earned enough credits to graduate with a high-school diploma at the age of sixteen.

Brad's career took off, and he trained or competed on the water in a kayak three hundred days each year. Off-seasons provided time for other pursuits, and Brad was anything but idle. His number-one priority became the development of First Descents, an organization offering free, weeklong trips in the outdoors for young adults with cancer. In 2001, at the age of nineteen, Brad was granted nonprofit status and was ready to take his first team of young adults out on the waters. All he needed was a group of clients who would believe in him and what he had to offer.

After his aunt's diagnosis, Brad had also worked at Eagle Mount, a therapeutic program providing recreational outdoor experiences for people with disabilities and children with cancer. When he was ready to take on his first group of kayaking cancer patients, Brad turned to his colleagues at Eagle Mount, asking if any of their patients might want to give his program a try. He had gained some added credibility when Nike had signed on as a First Descent sponsor, but he was still a nineteen-year-old asking already vulnerable people to follow him out into the backcountry for a week. Ultimately, through Eagle Mount, Brad found fifteen takers for that first expedition. As he looks back now in amazement that it actually went off without a hitch, he realizes that this group was the first to launch his dream. Many others would follow on the river with Brad and the good people who have since joined him at First Descents.

One of Brad's longtime friends is Kelly Starrett, a physical therapist and owner of CrossFit San Francisco and the website mobilitywod. com. Years ago, Kelly, who was once a serious whitewater rafter and kayaker, had discovered CrossFit and turned Brad on to its methodology. After the two worked out together in Brad's garage gym for over six years, Kelly encouraged Brad to join a CrossFit affiliate, which he did in 2010, incorporating the program into his kayaking training.

Now the CEO of First Descents, a thriving nonprofit organization, Brad is somewhat awestruck by what has evolved. He remembers the slow times in the first three years when the program involved a

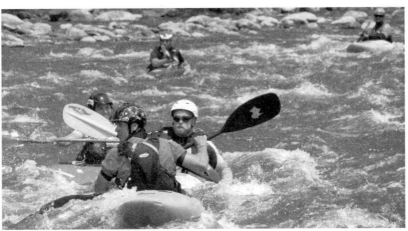

Brad Ludden and Neil Taylor, Colorado River, Colorado.

mere one to three weeks of "camps" each year. After that, though, "the fire caught and it just blew up. We knew people would like it, but it's a really big step to ask them to challenge themselves in this major way when they're already going through cancer." Brad was admittedly naïve about certain aspects of liability in the initial phases, but this allowed him to forge ahead and get the ball rolling in ways he might not have had he been privy to all the legal barriers. Now, First Descents has an active advisory board and a standard, formal process to address the many legal and medical issues relevant to taking cancer patients and survivors on outdoor adventures.

The First Descents model is simple: Take a group of young adults—ages eighteen to thirty-nine—outdoors for a week, teach them necessary skills in a certain sport or activity, help them apply those skills in small ways, and conclude with a culminating, significant and serious adventure challenge. The group might kayak extreme rapids, or climb a mountain peak, or tackle a particularly hairy rock climb. Completing these challenges alongside others who share their experience of cancer allows something powerful to occur. There are the transformative psychological effects for the individuals, including a great sense of accomplishment, increased self-confidence, a strong feeling of efficacy and control, and the elation that comes with a realization that life can go on after cancer. Beyond the impact on the individual, a greater force is at work during camp at First Descents: a community is formed within days. With no formal process in place for the unfolding of relationships among the campers, nonetheless, or perhaps because of this lack of structure, the bonds do develop. And the relationships are meaningful and lasting.

The campers are provided with an opportunity to be with others who have also had to accept a scary diagnosis, endure painful treatments, survive operations, and manage life—in some cases after disfiguring surgery. For many, it is the first time since their diagnosis that they have socialized and connected with other cancer patients their age. They can talk openly about their experiences and feelings.

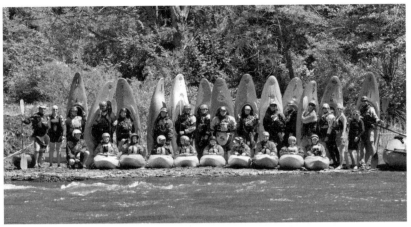

First Descents group in Hood River, Oregon.

They can discuss hair loss, embarrassing bathroom problems, low blood counts, and other side effects of chemotherapy and radiation. They can talk about the struggles of raising kids while nauseated, looking for work while fatigued, or dating after losing both breasts. They can leave behind their identity as the "one" with cancer while creating a new identity as a cancer survivor, one of many, part of a group of peers.

According to Brad, the young adult population of cancer patients is largely disconnected and underserved compared with other demographics. Pediatric cancer patients are part of a widely acknowledged population whose needs are addressed time and again with programs and research focused on them. Similarly, geriatric cancer receives significant attention in our medical world—from research to care—and everything in between. While these services are critical and greatly appreciated, part of Brad's mission is to bring the same attention and focus to young adults with cancer who, in addition to coping with a serious diagnosis, are also often facing significant life challenges when the disease strikes. His contribution of First Descents speaks volumes about the need for this population to be integrated into a community and to receive psychosocial care that recognizes and addresses their unique set of concerns.

From the moment they arrive on-site, all campers at First Descents are given nicknames; their real names are not used at all throughout the week. At first just a gimmick, this practice developed as standard procedure when it became clear to Brad and his staff that the nicknames allow campers to inhabit a new self and create an identity of their choosing, which may or may not have to do with their status as a cancer patient. As the clients embark on this life-changing experience, the nicknames become associated with something new and positive. According to Brad, "The nickname is not cancer. It's not bills. It's not illness. It's like nicknames in the military or the customary trail name one is given after hiking the Pacific Crest or Appalachian Trail. That name is a new self, a new opportunity. It allows them to create something different."

As a psychologist, I was interested in First Descents' attempt to incorporate a structured therapy component within the program. Apparently, instead of fostering discussion, it had the unintended effect of shutting down the campers. They did not like being forced to share their feelings about having cancer. Instead, with no psychologists in the field and no structured forum for discussion, the process unfolds organically and works, in large part, because of the bonding effects of the rigorous outdoor challenges. Brad explains:

> *We can all relate to how you connect with people when you are out in nature doing something challenging—your lives are in each other's hands. You connect with people with whom you've shared real life experiences and challenges. It's not like just going out to a bar with a group of buddies. ... Anything based on a legitimate challenge will draw a tight community. There is something bonding about sharing in success, vulnerability, fear, adrenaline, and accomplishment, all of which come through a challenge. ... You take that closeness—that bond—*

and multiply it by about two hundred. It's a whole other level of connection, because they all also have cancer.

Brad emphasizes the importance of the "legitimacy" of the challenges the First Descent campers conquer. The challenge experience is transformative primarily and specifically because it is difficult and intense. "We don't dumb this down for cancer," he says. "When you get to the bottom of that last rapid, or to the top of that climb, you're going to be like, *'holy shit, I just did something impressive. Cancer does not define my life.'* It restores a lot of the psychosocial damage caused by cancer. It leads to self-confidence, a sense of control. We give them a challenge they can control and win tangibly. Cancer is not something they can control ... but no one can take that summit away from them." Sharing the summit with other survivors makes the culminating experience that much more meaningful and integrated.

Brad, now an avid CrossFitter, draws many parallels with CrossFit, First Descents, and his outdoor pursuits:

Much like CrossFit, I find community in each sport or outdoor activity I partake in. There is a bond and respect among outdoorsmen. Whether ... I'm riding in Moab with my biking buddies, or spending a week on a river with my paddling buddies, it's always like family. ... When you meet a fellow CrossFitter, there's an immediate level of mutual respect and understanding that's hard to find anywhere else. Additionally, I find a lot of support from my friends at CrossFit outside of the gym. They always show up to my events, we all recreate together, and if someone needs a hand, you can count on a CrossFitter to be there. It's more than a workout and more than a gym. It's a language that only we speak. I believe that through challenge, we grow closer. Any time you challenge yourself in a group, you bond strongly with the others. You share an achievement, whether it's ... navigating class-five rapids, or completing Fran [a signature CrossFit workout]— you can relate to each other on a unique and legitimate level. One of the main reasons First Descents works to heal the psychosocial effects of cancer is because we put a group of strangers through a legitimate challenge, and they immediately bond. ... To me, the most striking thing is just how close that challenge draws you to others. You learn so much about the people you're with as well as yourself and, afterwards, you all have a story to tell that is your own.

As it turns out, the connection with other campers and the community experience is what is treasured most by First Descent clients. They tend to maintain contact with their First Descent friends for years after camp, despite geographic distances. Technology helps immensely in this effort; each camp group has its own Google group, many of whom are alive and thriving up to five years after the community was originally created out in the field. Facebook is also helpful, and Brad points out that many First Descent alums use a shot from their culminating challenge at First Descents as their Facebook profile picture.

First Descents clients are invited to come back to camp up to three times. After that, they are encouraged to take on a physical competition outside of the program as a fund-raising effort to "pay it forward" and allow another camper to attend. These challenges include marathons, triathlons, bike rides, adventure races, and the like. The community thus grows from within through the tenacity and generosity of those who have benefited themselves. Here again, we see the power of altruism in a community where goodness thrives and real human connections are made, growing out of a psychological need for support and understanding.

The Tale of Tailz

Neil Taylor completed his first camp at First Descents in 2009, just over a year after he was diagnosed with a malignant brain tumor. At the time, Neil was a teacher and soccer coach at the Greenwood School in Putney, Vermont. Greenwood is a boarding school for boys ages nine to fourteen who are diagnosed with a variety of learning disabilities and attention problems. Neil loved his job and was a favorite with the boys at Putney. A self-described "adrenaline junkie," Neil lived in Costa Rica for five months after high school, graduated from college, worked in Alta, Utah, where he could ski all he wanted and was now ready to be near home and begin living a more rooted existence.

In 2008, Neil's girlfriend became concerned when he was experiencing tunnel vision in his left eye for bouts of about three to four seconds at a time, before his vision would return to normal. Although Neil was inclined to think that he just needed more sleep, his girlfriend insisted that he see a doctor. An MRI revealed that Neil had a tumor the size of an orange in the left hemisphere of his brain. Doctors were amazed that Neil could even walk and talk, given the severity, size, and location of the tumor. Neil found it disturbing that each doctor who read his films was more in awe than the one before. There was little time for Neil and his family to decide where he should undergo the necessary brain surgery, let alone process the devastating information they were receiving. After frenetic research, they decided on a hospital in New Hampshire, and the surgery was scheduled.

The plan was for doctors to keep Neil semiconscious throughout the operation so that they could elicit feedback from him while they removed parts of his brain. Unfortunately, while in the hospital the night before his scheduled surgery, Neil went into massive seizures, necessitating full sedation and a totally different surgical procedure. Instead of removing 90 percent of the tumor as planned, doctors could only remove 70 percent. They also had less control over the effects of the surgery.

When Neil woke up from the operation and opened his eyes, he couldn't see a thing and did not know if it was night or day. He was not informed or did not realize that one of the possible complications of his surgery was blindness. His hands and feet were tied down and zipped into restraints; apparently, he had put up quite a fight to remove the oxygen tube from his throat. Neil can laugh now, recalling how the nurses told him they had never seen such a fighter. Neil now knows that it was the pressure on his optic nerve that caused him to go blind. His eyes were perfectly healthy, but his optic nerve was shot. He hasn't seen a thing since.

Neil remembers being "totally despondent" those first few days in the hospital. "When someone came into my room from the Vermont Institute for the Blind, I didn't hear a fucking word they had to say. There was a possibility in the first three months that my sight would return. I was banking on that. I thought in my heart that I couldn't be a blind person. Turns out the people at Vermont Institute for the Blind have been my saviors ever since. They fund everything for me and buy me adaptable tools. They've been great." But, in those early days, Neil was not open to help, and it would take some time before he could accept his new reality. "The months passed, and I had to become resigned to the fact that I was blind. Which is one of the biggest losses you can have in your life."

After Neil's initial recovery from surgery, he endured a full year of treatments, including chemotherapy and radiation. He remembers being completely fatigued and "out of it" much of the time. Forced to move in with his parents, he recalls how that was "a huge regression, hard in and of itself." Once Neil had recovered from his treatments, he moved on to a four-month stay at the Carroll Center in Massachusetts, a nonprofit facility where blind and visually impaired people learn to live independently through rehabilitation, skills training, and adaptive technologies. Because he was a Vermont resident, Neil's stay at

Carroll was funded by the Vermont Institute for the Blind; he was entitled to four months at the Carroll Center, while Massachusetts residents were capped at six weeks when state funding expired. Neil was extremely grateful for his time there since he learned how to get around with a cane, how to cook, pay bills, shop, use the Internet, how to entertain himself, and myriad other independent-living skills.

Upon graduation from the Carroll Center, Neil moved into an apartment in Brattleboro, Vermont, approximately thirty minutes from his parents' home. He still lives "right in the thick of it" in the city, and though the sound of trucks going by on the highway near his apartment was at first unsettling, he is now used to the noise.

In 2009, over a year after his diagnosis, Neil's friend, who himself had Hodgkin's lymphoma, connected Neil with Brad Ludden. Neil learned a bit about First Descents from Brad and was easily persuaded to give one of his kayak camps a try. Looking back on the opportunity and experience of his first camp, Neil—nicknamed Tailz—is emphatic about how much it changed his world:

I was thrilled, because so much of my life had disappeared. I'd always been an athlete and enjoyed doing crazy shit, but I couldn't do anything anymore. There was a huge void in my life. Everything is visual. I can't play darts, or throw the lacrosse ball with my dad, or hit a tennis ball with my mom, or enjoy art at the museum with my sister, or see the beautiful girl at the bar who isn't talking to anyone. I miss driving and getting in my car and just getting the fuck out of it. And I miss beautiful sunsets—natural beauty. But First Descents has really done a lot in filling that void. I used to be an athlete. I used to get really high from physical activity and that stopped once I went blind, until First Descents. Kayaking is awesome, because it's such a sensual sport. You feel with your hips and your legs which way the rapids are pulling you, and you need to keep a straight line.

Of course, First Descents is about far more than the physical challenges, and Neil has also benefited greatly from the relational and community components. During his experiences as a camper at First Descents, Neil found solace in connecting with other cancer patients. "We can talk about it, we can laugh about it, we can cry about it. That is so powerful. The six days you spend with your fellow campers totally transcends cancer. I made lifelong friends from six days of being out there. It's not just about kayaking or rock climbing, it's about making friendships that will last a lifetime."

Other life changes have happened for Neil since kayaking the rapids with the First Descents community. With the support of Brad and other staff and campers, he has been training to become a massage therapist. Still completing his required hands-on hours, Neil has worked at a number of First Descent camps as an in-house massage therapist. The new service has proven to be welcomed by the campers and staff alike. Neil's goal is to work for First Descents five months out of every year, and Brad is more than happy to have him on board.

Neil's most recent trip with First Descents was in Moab, Utah, a place he had visited before he became blind and where he was initially reluctant to return. In fact, he was agitated by the possibility and worried that it would be agony to be in such a beautiful place, unable to appreciate its visual power this time around. With Brad's encouragement, Neil relented and found himself back in Moab, surrounded by his new community. "It turns out it was spectacular. I thought I would be really sad to be there and not be able to see the arch, and it would be just like I'm standing in my kitchen. But I kept an open mind. It sounds trite, but certain senses become heightened and more acute when you lose your vision. Standing there, I felt the wind in my hair and I smelled the air and smelled the desert and felt the feeling. It felt so special that I didn't feel sad." Hearing Neil reflect on this Moab experience took my breath away. I asked Brad about it soon after, and he confirmed the enormity of the emotion wrapped up in that encounter.

Neil is extremely grateful for Brad and First Descents and the community they have brought into his life. "I'm just learning to deal with being blind and to get up every day and wake up happy and take on life. Things that I used to take for granted are real challenges for me. Every day I have to accept these challenges just to live my life. First Descents has really helped me with that. You meet these people who have had multiple fights with cancer. They are just strong people, and you know that because you went through a little bit of what they've been through." Neil also credits his family for their devotion, unconditional love and support, and for allowing him to live life as fully as possible.

While he does not sugarcoat his future and is quite candid about the limitations of his condition, Neil also keeps an incredibly positive perspective and continues to take on challenges and grab life by the horns. Indeed, at the time I first interviewed him, he was preparing for a forty-two-mile tandem bike ride with Brad through the five boroughs of New York City; Neil will peddle while Brad steers. They are doing this to raise money for another camper to attend First Descents.

Brad and Neil are obviously special people. In fact, my encounters with them both left me pondering a divine force at work in planting them in our midst. When their paths crossed, neither could have predicted the impact they would have on each other. Their connection is one part of a larger, fierce, and thriving community of survivors and compassionate, dedicated supporters. Their story is a touching example of the human spirit and the difference we can make, both as individuals and, more powerfully, as part of a community. I think we can agree that we can all use more Brad and Tailz in our lives.

Matt's Story

~

Matt's mother, Carole, was one of the first clients to walk into our gym back in 2002 when we were still calling it Personal Fitness of Marin. She trained in semiprivate sessions with TJ for over five years before he approached her with his idea of group workouts that he would call "The Metabolic." Reluctant at first to change to a group setting, Carole ultimately agreed to give it a try. She ended up surprising herself with how much she loved the workouts and the energy of the group. Over time, after The Metabolic became CrossFit and Carole was fully immersed in the TJ's Gym community, she began recruiting family members to join in the fun.

In January 2010, Carole's son, Matt, started our CrossFit program. He was out of shape, overweight, and hadn't exercised in years. The father of two teenagers who worked in his family business, Matt had let himself go for some time, focusing, instead, on the athletic pursuits of his son, a mountain biking star. Matt dove right into the workouts and the community, coming to classes three days a week and supplementing his CrossFit workouts with two days each week in our Barbell Club where he bettered his Olympic weightlifting skills. He took seriously TJ's nutrition advice and changed the way he ate and shopped for groceries. After five months as part of TJ's Gym, Matt had lost thirty pounds and looked and felt like a different person. His wife and son had also joined the community and were experiencing their own benefits and connection as part of something bigger than just a place to work out.

Within his first days of joining the gym, Matt appreciated the community environment at TJ's Gym. He recalls, "The unique thing that struck me right away about TJ's Gym was the people and the camaraderie everyone shared, regardless of their ability. It was very much a community like in Martial Arts, which I had studied previously. It was tight knit. I quickly made new friends and acquaintances who became almost motivators of their own to a degree. It was like a bunch of buddies you were accountable to, to support or give a rash of crap to if they didn't show."

In October, 2010, ten months after joining the gym, Matt was mountain biking with some friends in Downieville, California. He suffered a freak accident, falling off a cliff and plummeting sixty feet into the south fork of the Yuba River. He sat in the icy waters of the Yuba river for about ninety minutes before paramedics and rescue personnel arrived. Three hours passed from the time of the accident until they were able to get him out of the ravine to a place where a helicopter could evacuate him. When all was said and done, Matt had shattered his pelvis in six places, had broken nine ribs, had fractured his tailbone, and had punctured his left lung. He jokes that breaking his heel bone was the least of his injuries. Considering what could have happened to Matt, he feels lucky that his injuries were not worse, despite their severity and the extent to which he is still fighting to recover, a year later.

Matt feels that his workouts at TJ's Gym had saved his life: "I believe firmly that my physical conditioning played a huge part of minimizing the potential disastrous aftermath of the fall. Although the injuries were very serious, it could have been much worse. My core strength kept my internal organs protected and I sustained no injuries to them at all. My improved physical conditioning kept me alive in freezing water and evening freezing temperatures. My core temperature when I arrived at the hospital was eighty-eight degrees. I had no neck and shoulder injuries, due to all that core work ... and those damn thrusters!"

When word of Matt's accident spread, the people of TJ's Gym stepped up to help. Some organized dinner delivery schedules, some helped Matt's wife move furniture to the lower level of the house so Matt didn't have to climb the stairs, others sent cards and emails on a regular basis. "It is an act of kindness that still chokes me up to this day," Matt says, months after the incident. For a while, though, even with all the support he was receiving, Matt struggled with the

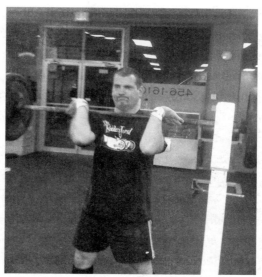

Matt Taylor at TJ's Gym before his accident.

recovery process. He was confined to a wheelchair, taking pain medication "around the clock. The combination of confinement and medication was unbearable. ... It was killing me not to be able to go back into TJs' and work out with my gang. My buddy took me to watch my Barbell Club group one Sunday when I was moving around better, and that felt awesome. Just watching my group working out was a great motivator to rehab as quickly and thoroughly as possible and rebuild my fitness level."

Unfortunately, Matt's recovery has not gone smoothly. Though he has re-entered the gym and worked out intermittently, his body has not cooperated, and for now at least Matt is unable to participate. He is proud of his wife whose dedication to the program, combined with her natural athletic talents, has allowed her to optimize her fitness. He admits that his son is now stronger than he is, while his daughter is discovering the benefits of her newfound strength on the soccer field. Clearly Matt is still part of the community, and even though he cannot participate physically at the moment, the relationships remain:

I think for me being part of a community like TJ's has enhanced my experience of returning to fitness. You have people that share in your small victories and support you in your setbacks or plateaus. It may be nothing more than a pat on the back after a metcon [metabolic conditioning] beat-down, but to know that others, friends, are there suffering along with you towards a common goal makes a huge difference for me. ... A traditional gym setting ... is an isolating type of experience. Unless you are an extremely self-motivating personality type, you are pretty much on your own. There is very little interaction with others working out. ... My entire family's participation in CrossFit has been very rewarding and allows us another connection or bond, as a family.

Matt hopes to be back in the gym some day, but for now, he continues to feel connected to the community with its sustaining support.

Chapter 8

The Military Community

As you've gathered by now, one of the reasons the CrossFit program lends itself so naturally and organically to the building of communities is the common ground of experiences shared by its members. If you CrossFit with regularity, you know what it means to allow yourself to be vulnerable among peers, to push to physical limits on a consistent basis, and to make sacrifices in order to improve your fitness. You know that the intensity of a workout matters and that true fitness does not result from exercising while reading a magazine. You know that working toward your goals requires significant effort and change and that the process is not easy. You also appreciate the fun and humor shared along the way, which keeps you coming back for more. While working out at a CrossFit gym, people get to know each other and friendships are born and nurtured. Even strangers whose paths cross out in the world tend to feel a sense of kinship based on the simple fact that they are CrossFitters.

This kind of shared experience leading to a sense of connection is not unique to CrossFitters. As we've explored, many individuals with strong religious affiliations feel connected to others who practice and believe as part of a faith-based community. Similarly, wilderness adventurers and survivalists often have a palpable sense of kinship, knowing they have tempted fate and weathered the demands of nature. Olympic athletes might have a comparable experience, understanding that they have devoted significant portions of their lives to training and competing, and that each has managed the pressures of elite athleticism. Athletes who push themselves during fund-raisers in support of a special cause find a similar camaraderie and bond.

Perhaps the most powerful connection occurs among those who have served in the military. If you have gone to battle in the armed forces of your country, you are bound to feel connection with others who have done the same. As a civilian psychologist lacking this direct experience, I can only approximate what that bond is all about. Life in the trenches involves intense situations at physical, emotional, hormonal, and interpersonal levels so life-altering, even life-threatening, that they are natural building blocks for bonding with others. As Shakespeare's King Henry V states so eloquently before the Battle of Agincourt: "We few, we happy few, we band of brothers: For he today that sheds his blood with me shall be my brother."[37] Reliance on others for life-saving backup in a combat situation provides a unique and heightened connection. Families of military personnel share their own brand of community, understanding the challenges of having a loved one in service.

The United States military has a well-established community of its own, with numerous organizations dedicated to providing and maintaining a support network for families of those who serve. The lives of military families are often interrupted with constant location changes along with the uncertainty and risk of service abroad, and through the ultimate sacrifice when loved ones are lost in battle.

Historically, CrossFit has had a strong relationship with the United States military. One of the initial aims of CrossFit founder, Greg Glassman, was to utilize his program to raise the fitness levels of our country's defenders. Over the years, CrossFit has donated many thousands of dollars of equipment to the U.S. military, both domestically and abroad, in order to help military personnel maintain a CrossFit routine. The power of the CrossFit community has served the needs of military personnel and their families through fund-raising efforts for wounded soldiers and the families of fallen heroes. CrossFit coaches have also worked with veterans to develop and maintain fitness programs, often helping them deal with significant, traumatic injuries. There are compelling stories to be told about the interaction between the CrossFit community and U.S. military personnel. What follows is a small sampling of these stories.

The Disposable Heroes Project: Another Brad Gives Back—with Passion and Commitment

One day in July of 2009, Brad McKee watched a story on Fox News about Keith Zeier, a wounded veteran who was hit by an improvised explosive device (IED) while serving in Iraq in 2006. Shrapnel had severed his leg, and he also suffered a brain injury. He was told he would never walk again. After numerous surgeries and endless painkillers to maintain some level of comfort, this battle veteran was back on his feet, defying the odds. Keith decided to run 100 miles to raise awareness of, and funds for, wounded veterans throughout the United States. He collapsed at mile seventy-five, but after refusing to be taken to the hospital, Keith finished the run, raising over $60,000 for the Special Operations Warrior Foundation.

Brad, a former Marine Corps sergeant, was deeply moved by Keith's story. That night, at a bar with a childhood friend, Samuel Macaluso, Brad vowed that he, too, would run 100 miles in support of wounded veterans and in memory of fallen heroes. "Seeing that story on the news triggered a promise I had made to myself when I got out of the Marine Corps—to do something for these guys who continually serve us, for our wounded veterans and fallen troops."

The next day, Brad and Sam traded ideas about how to create an identity for their project. They landed on the name Disposable Heroes Project (DHP), one close to home for Brad. Many of the marines with whom he had served had a tattoo of a black flag across their chest to signify their willingness to do anything it takes to serve their country and provide freedom for all of us, including the ultimate sacrifice. Brad sees this as the "positive" angle of the disposable heroes term. The negative side for Brad is how the media can make our troops appear disposable by glossing over their deaths in a quick sound bite, or by reducing them to a number. Brad is passionate about his cause: "Every day that the media considers our troops to be just a number, or the general population forgets about them, they become disposable; we have to be sure that never happens."

Although the DHP officially started in August of 2009, the real kick-off event was Brad's 100-mile run in April of 2010. A number of wounded veterans joined Brad at the start of the race in Hammond, Louisiana, including a double-amputee from Florida who was driven there by the medic who had saved his life in combat. Accompanying Brad on different portions of the run were wounded veterans, marines with whom he had served in Iraq, family, friends, and members of the New Orleans Saints professional football team. Brad drew heavily from the inspiration of these individuals during his run, especially the last twenty miles when he ran alongside Corporal G. Corporal Isaac Gallegos and Brad had met at the San Antonio Burn Center where Brad had begun cultivating relationships with wounded veterans being treated there. Another victim of an IED in Iraq, Corporal G suffered from burns over seventy-five-percent of his body, including his face. Despite doctors' warnings to avoid sweating because of lost sweat glands, Isaac ran the final stretch of Brad's run with him, to the cheers and tears of hundreds of supporters along the route.

Despite nagging injuries, Brad finished his run as planned, building momentum for the Disposable Heroes Project. His only training prior to the run had been with CrossFit workouts. He had learned the hard way that endurance training involving miles and miles of running did not work for his body. When he had trained for marathons in the past, he had experienced significant knee problems and other overuse injuries. He had run the Marine Corps Marathon with two aching knees, limping each step past mile fifteen, persevering because he had told the wife of a fallen marine with whom he'd served in Iraq that he would run the race with her in memory of her husband. Later, he ran the New York City Marathon with Keith Zeier, the same injured veteran who had run the hundred-mile race that inspired Brad in the first place. Brad wore a fifty-pound pack this time, to mimic the efforts of soldiers who travel with heavy gear. Unfortunately, his knee locked up during the first mile of the marathon, forcing him to walk the whole distance. He finished five seconds before the eight-hour cutoff time. With those experiences behind him, Brad chose to train for his hundred-mile race using only CrossFit workouts. He believes that CrossFit provides the best functional fitness possible, and his body responded with a decrease in injuries and an ability to sustain effort throughout the hundred-mile event.

Carey Peterson, a reporter for the *CrossFit Journal,* captured the emotion and power of Brad's journey in a four-part video series in the online journal. During an interview with Carey prior to his run, Brad shared some thoughts as he anticipated the struggles he might face along the way:

I've already programmed in my mind ... if I start feeling that pain, which I know I will, I'm going to think about the reason I'm running a hundred miles. ... My motivation is these wounded veterans and these fallen heroes. And some of these wounded vets will be running with me. So if I'm hurting and I look to my left or to my right and I have a wounded veteran running with me, knowing the sacrifices he's made for his country, I don't think there's any way I can say: "Hey, you know what? You as a wounded veteran keep on going. I have to stop." I just don't see it happening, no matter how much pain I'm in.[38]

With the 100-mile race behind him and significant publicity in its wake, Brad knew that the Disposable Heroes Project had legs. Its mission is broad: Brad and his partners seek to help wounded veterans and the families of fallen heroes "in any way possible, by any means possible. If there's a need out there and someone brings it to our attention, we're ready to make it happen." It's something like a Make-a-Wish Foundation for the wounded veteran/fallen hero population. Brad cultivates relationships with those in need and finds

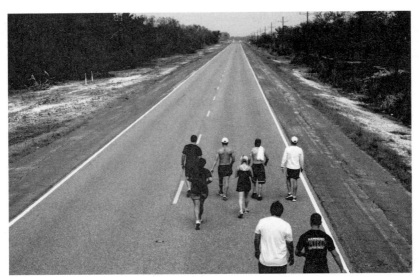

Brad McKee's 100-mile run to raise money for the Disposable Heroes Project.

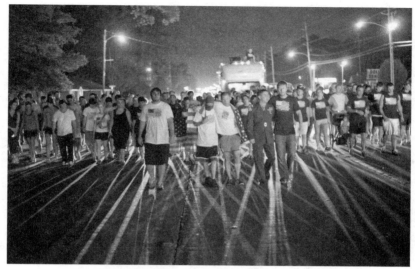

***Brad McKee and Isaac Gallegos at the end of the
100-mile run in Hammond, LA.***

out how he can brighten the day of a veteran or provide assistance to
the family of a fallen hero.

Funds must be raised to sustain the program, and the DHP does
so primarily in two ways: Their most significant source of income is
through the sale of their T-shirts online. The DHP's second largest
source of revenue comes from fund-raisers held at CrossFit gyms
around the country, bringing people together for an intense, brutal
workout. Participants donate money and are inspired by Brad's
preworkout speech about finding motivation when the going gets
tough. He encourages people to think about the men and women who
have sacrificed for our country. There is rarely a dry eye in the crowd,
and every individual gives maximum effort, pushing harder than they
ever have.

One such fund-raiser was held in April 2011 in Warr Acres,
Oklahoma, where athletes from twelve different CrossFit affiliates
came together in solidarity to support the project. Prior to the event,
Brad had contacted the family of Army Staff Sergeant Jack M. Martin
III, who was killed by an IED on September 29, 2009, in Jolo Island,

Philippines. CrossFit has a practice of naming specific workouts for fallen heroes and "Jack" is one such workout. When the workouts are posted on the CrossFit website, there is a picture of the hero and a brief blurb about his service, his family, and his death.

While Brad believes that this is a great start in honoring fallen heroes, he would like to see more information about each soldier made available to the public; part of his mission is to bring to life these men and women who have made the ultimate sacrifice. "Every hero workout is one too many. CrossFit is a close-knit community, and we already spout off the names of hero workouts all the time and know exactly what we're talking about. But hopefully we can post the name and know exactly what that guy was like, what he liked to do, what kind of person he was. It will put a lot more meaning and emotion into the workout." His goal is to meet and interview every family of every hero for whom CrossFit has named a workout. Online visitors to the website would then be able to click on a link for each posted workout, learning more about its namesake through memories and anecdotes of loved ones. Brad is committed to moving forward with these bios, and given his experience with the family of Jack Martin III, he knows that the result will be well worth the effort.

Jack's family welcomed Brad into their home the night before the DHP workout to be held in his honor. They shared stories about who Jack was, about his personality and his sense of humor. They agreed to let Brad wear Jack's medic pack during the workout in order to have his presence felt, and they expressed their desire to finally see Jack's remains. It seems that when Jack was killed, his parents flew to Washington State to be with Jack's widow, but at the time his remains had not yet been transported. Since then, Jack's ashes were brought to his wife, and his parents wanted to make the trip back to Washington. Through the DHP, Brad was able to work with Southwest Airlines and get tickets for Jack's parents to fly to Washington at their convenience.

Brad is quick to point out that one of the things people respect most about the Disposable Heroes Project is that it is run entirely by unpaid volunteers. While project money does cover Brad's airfare when he travels, he has yet to stay in a hotel, preferring to bunk on someone's floor so that more money can be put toward the DHP mission. This selfless dedication is typical of Brad; he learned at an early age to be gritty and strong in the face of adversity. His parents divorced when he was six years old and Brad, the oldest of three children, felt an immediate responsibility and sense of duty. He felt the absence of his father, despite occasional weekend visits, and "had no choice but to grow up faster. [The visits] didn't take the place of having a father figure in the house seven days a week. I learned real quick how to make decisions and how to have confidence in those decisions and be the man of the house at a very young age."

Brad credits his mom for the job she did raising him and his siblings as a single parent. His strong religious faith also helped guide him through his childhood and beyond, and he maintains that faith at present. Brad's experience playing high school sports—football, baseball, and soccer—helped him cultivate his leadership skills, encouraging other athletes to join in a common goal. With these early leadership experiences internalized, Brad's role as a marine sniper became a natural outlet for their expression:

> Once I joined the Marine Corps and became a sniper, that's a whole other level of competence and leadership. ... I was twenty-one-years old when I graduated from sniper school. To be able to take a team of six guys to Iraq that you're in charge of at the age of twenty-one, you really have no other option but to grow up fast. I think there's an age limit set on too many things in this world—"you have you be older to do this," or "just wait, you're moving too fast." I don't think I'm moving too fast at all.

Still, Brad recognizes that there are things that are important for him to do, even while he pursues his commitment to the DHP. He completed one year of college prior to enlisting in the Marine Corps, realizing that the classroom "wasn't my spot," and soon found himself deployed in Iraq as a sniper. During his four years of active duty, Brad served in Iraq twice. When he left the Corps, he was forced to reckon with what he wanted to do with the rest of his life. He did not want to become a law enforcement officer as many of his fellow veterans did, but decided to return to college at Louisiana State University, where he studied for another eighteen months. It was during this time that Brad started the DHP and was introduced to CrossFit by a friend. Almost immediately, Brad was hooked, so much so that he decided to open his own CrossFit affiliate. The significant challenges of attending college, running his own business, and creating and managing the DHP drove Brad to reevaluate his studies, and he has chosen to pursue his final college credits via Internet courses. Asked why he perseveres with his studies as a successful business owner and philanthropic champion, Brad highlights a promise he had made to his mother:

I promised myself and my mother that I would finish college. ... I thought it was important, no matter what I decided to do, that I have a college degree just in case things do fall in the wrong direction. It's also good when you raise your kids to tell them you have a college education, so you set the example. It's important for me to finish it out.

Brad is a man of his word. The other big promise he has kept is the one he made to himself when leaving the Marine Corps behind: "I told myself that if I got out I would continually serve these guys. ... It's something that I promised myself I would do, and I'll keep that promise and I'll fight until the day I die for the guys who are serving our country." The Disposable Heroes Project is Brad's fulfillment of this promise, and it has delivered in so many meaningful ways. Brad is proud of efforts like taking a depressed wounded veteran on a tour of Boston Harbor and Fenway Park or helping a double-amputee keep his housing despite being unable to hold a job and pay his rent.

Brad is passionate about maintaining relationships with the people he has helped, since part of the point is to keep them engaged and let them know they are not forgotten. Brad has been touched by the willingness of families to speak with him about their loved ones, realizing how reluctant they often are to talk to outsiders, especially when media coverage is involved. His own standing as a former Marine Corps sniper gives him significant credibility with these families, and for good reason. Brad gets their experience at a level that would not be possible had he never served in Iraq. As an insider in the military community, Brad meets with them annually at the gravesite of one of their fallen brothers. He also knows how military community contacts and support groups helped his own mother during his tours in Iraq. Reflecting on this, Brad made what I found to be a simple, yet poignant comment about our desire for connection: "Military support groups are filled with people like all others. Everyone wants to find a group of people to connect with who have been through the same thing they have."

Brad has his own ideas about how to run the DHP. While he understands the bureaucratic requirements of operating an official nonprofit, he is sometimes frustrated by people who advise him to be politically correct, to have a detailed mission statement, or to have every detail of the project planned in advance. Brad explains:

> *This kind of planning is great. But when you are trying to help wounded veterans and the families of fallen troops, the needs often change. So when I say whatever the needs are we get 'em done, that's exactly what I mean. That's why our mission statement is broad. We had a meeting last night and we talked about what happens if a guy is killed and his daughter is so down in the dumps that the little girl might need a trip to Disneyworld. We'll just do it. Or for a wounded*

veteran, it could be anything from buying a prosthetic leg if the government doesn't cover it, to taking him out to a baseball game to let him know that people still do care. The suicide rate for returning veterans is just outrageous, and there are things we can do to let them know that we care about them and haven't forgot them.

Through Brad's contacts and the Disposable Heroes Project, a vast and dedicated community continues to grow. It is a community committed to helping those in need and keeping alive the memories of those who have sacrificed their lives for our country. Brad draws parallels between DHP and CrossFit Inc. He highlights CrossFit's approach to their affiliate community, allowing affiliate owners to operate independently. He cites their small staff, low overhead, and the simplicity of the physical plants housing their operations. "Greg Glassman just gets the job done. He addresses the critical needs. He is unlike others in the fitness industry." Brad also notes how DHP and CrossFit both cut to the chase and follow through on their aims, without a whole lot of pomp and circumstance. "We each have one goal. We at the DHP are raising awareness of wounded veterans and fallen heroes, and CrossFit is getting people fit. We both get straight to it and address the needs of our populations."

Disposable Hero: Corporal G

Isaac Gallegos was, in many ways, destined to be a marine. His father was a marine and Isaac was born at Camp Lejeune, a Marine Corps base in North Carolina. As a single father of four, his dad was not permitted to take on a Marine duty stationed overseas, and he eventually left the service in the early 1990s. Isaac's father remarried when Isaac was four, so in addition to occasional visits with his biological mother during the summer, he had a steady mother figure in his stepmother. The family moved around a great deal during Isaac's early years when his father was in the military. When he left the marines, Isaac's dad became a police officer in Los Angeles, where the family lived for some time, though they continued to move over the years.

Isaac recalls that his choice to become a marine seemed a natural one, following his father's example, but he also had other reasons and individuals influencing his decision:

> *My dad being a marine had a strong influence on me becoming one, but I also worked with a few marines when I was in community college. I understood how they worked and how they operated, and it gave me a better idea of which branch of the military I would choose. I liked the camaraderie, the brothership. I liked the way they go out there and do the job, without pissing off the people, the natives, and they're going to try and do it without casualties if they can.*

Isaac trained at Camp Pendleton and was six months into serving his first tour of active duty in 2006 when his life was changed forever: He was another victim of a pressure-plate IED explosion in Iraq. Seventy-five percent of his body was burned, his jaw was shattered, and his left hand was fractured. He was flown to various locations en route from Iraq to his eventual destination at Brooke Army Medical Center in San Antonio, Texas. Isaac was twenty-one years old. He spent six months at the burn center where he was treated, enduring multiple surgeries. After his release from the hospital, he lived off-base and returned to Brooke for surgery and therapy from time to time. Isaac's father and stepmother moved to San Antonio for a few years to help take care of him, for which he is deeply grateful.

Even now, five years later, Isaac still suffers from the traumatic effects of his injuries. His face is disfigured, his elbows cannot fully extend, and he is strictly limited in outdoor activities, under doctor's orders, because of the dangers of exposure to the sun. Isaac recalls that the most challenging time for him was the recovery period after he had been on bed rest following several surgeries. It took him three years to become somewhat active again, including the ability to go for an occasional outdoor run. Ultimately, he participated in the run of his life when he ran the last twenty miles of Brad McKee's 100-mile run alongside Brad. Isaac remembers the emotions of the finish as if it were yesterday. He was overwhelmed by the number of people from the town of Hammond who came out to cheer them on as they finished the run. "The ending was just really nice," he says quietly. "It was emotional. … It was amazing."

Brad and Isaac had met through a mutual friend at the San Antonio burn center when Isaac was an inpatient. Brad had contacted the burn unit on behalf of the Disposable Heroes Project to see if any of the patients there could benefit from DHP resources. He was introduced to Isaac and the two got to chatting about Brad's 100-mile challenge which was planned for the following year. Isaac was intrigued and said he'd be happy to run with Brad, as long as surgery didn't interfere with the timing of the run.

Isaac is thankful for Brad and the DHP. In support of Brad's idea that wounded warriors are more likely to connect with others who have served than with outsiders, Isaac comments,

I like the DHP more than some of the other organizations, because they are personally involved. Family members and friends are nice to have, but when you have somebody who has gone through some of the same stuff, it's totally different. They've helped me, and if they ever need help from me, I'll be there for them. I'm doing great and don't need any help now, so I've told them to give anything I might get to the next guy in need. The help I got was friendship, support, and networking.

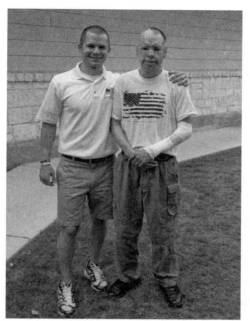

Brad McKee and Isaac Gallegos .

Indeed, one of the appeals of the Marines for Isaac was the culture within. "A lot of it has to do with history, traditions, and customs. They teach you that if the guy next you, to the side of you, behind you is a marine, he's your family and you don't ever forget that. When you're out there and all hell's breaking loose, he's going to be there for you and you're going to be there for him. In many ways you're closer than real family." It is this kind of culture—this kind of bond— that nurtures the DHP and fuels the vast network of groups to help our fallen troops.

After his initial recovery, Isaac slowly worked his way back to his job with the Marines. "I started bugging people to get out of there (the barracks), trying to return to a unit of the fleet, until they finally set me up here at Camp Pendleton." He is now an instructor for the School of Infantry, the SOI, for advanced infantry trainers and infantry training battalions. "It's not bad right now. It'll get me where I need to go and where I need to be. It's a progression." Isaac is on permanent light-duty status, so he is not able to participate in strenuous training. With over a year before his contract in the Marines ends, he is considering all options for what lies ahead. Asked to reflect on his choice to serve as a marine, given the toll it has taken on his body and his life, Isaac explained, "I have no regrets. No regrets. Can't regret anything you've done. All you can do is learn from it and see if you made any mistakes and don't do it again. We all go through periods of anger, but nothing that would ever stop me from doing anything I've wanted to get done."

At a makeshift ceremony at the end of his 100-mile run with Corporal G at his side, Brad McKee gave a short speech to the crowd, one he has used as a source of inspiration for the Disposable Heroes Project and for his CrossFit community, concluding with this thought: "When you go through life and you think you have obstacles in your way, think about guys like Isaac."

Scott Heintz and 9Line LLC

When ground forces in the United States Army need help with a wounded warrior, a medevac request is initiated. The procedure is called the 9Line request, since there are nine bits of information the ground forces relay to the medevac crew before they launch for the recovery of the wounded soldier or soldiers. Information includes the level of safety for landing, how many are wounded, severity of injuries, and other data valuable for the rescue mission.

During his twenty-six years as a medevac pilot in the United States Army, Scott Heintz was the recipient of countless 9Line requests, and he saw his share of drama and trauma in combat. He now runs a small business whose name is 9Line LLC. In contract with the United States Special Operations Command Care Coalition (USSOCOM) and funded by the Department of Defense, 9Line's purpose is to provide advocacy and support to America's seriously wounded Special Operations Forces and their families. The company is comprised mostly of retired senior military leaders whose careers centered on the management of the welfare of other warriors and their families. Together, these veterans have hundreds of years of experience providing support to members of our armed forces in combat, and they are now serving a similar function for wounded warriors reentering the world after a service disability.

Military personnel returning home after deployment face a wide spectrum of challenges, even when they are not physically injured. The psychological impact of immersion in combat is significant and well documented, and Hollywood has explored this aspect of war and its aftermath repeatedly over the years. Experiencing the stressors of the battlefield takes a great human toll, and many returning warriors find themselves exhausted, depressed, and introspective, suffering from posttraumatic stress and, in many cases, with suicidal thoughts. When a traumatic physical injury is added to the mix, homecoming is fraught with serious complications and obstacles. The spectrum of war wounds is horrific, from severe burns to loss of limbs to traumatic brain injuries. While well-intentioned family members may step up to help, they are often ill-equipped to manage the complex emotional needs of wounded warriors, to navigate the health care system or

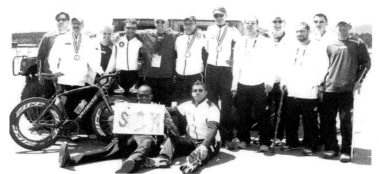

Scott Heintz, second row, fifth from left, at the 2011 Wounded Warrior Games with the "SOF Bionic Warriors" representing the U.S. Special Operations Command.

access valuable resources. Frequently, relatives are, themselves, traumatized by the altered status of the person they sent off to war, and they too are in need of support and treatment.

Recognizing the needs of this growing population of returning veterans, a number of organizations have been created—both private nonprofit and government funded. One such group is 9Line, providing basic support for wounded warriors through its Advocacy Program. The seven specially selected and trained 9Line advocates from across the country—all retired Special Forces, Command sergeant majors, or Medical Command sergeant majors—develop relationships with military personnel and their families, connecting them with the resources necessary for their physical well-being and emotional stability. Ideally, each advocate would be responsible for up to fifteen individuals, but as Scott Heintz points out, the service is "running more like a one-to-twenty or even one-to-twenty-five ratio, because of the number of injured."

The next level of assistance provided by 9Line is its Mentorship Program. Scott and his coworkers have identified approximately 100 Special Operations troops who, according to Scott, "are far enough along in the process of recovery that they can offer some beneficial insight to newly wounded warriors and their families in terms of what they can expect, what worked for them, the highs and lows they saw on their journey." Mentors are all unpaid volunteers and eighty percent of them have been on the receiving end of 9Line's services in the past. With their shared experience of having faced dark times, severe injury, and ongoing disability, they are in a unique position to help others down the long road of re-immersion into civilian life. Ninety-nine percent of mentors are veterans, but Scott has reached outside the military in order to find an appropriate mentor for a specific need. Once, for example, when Scott needed a mentor for a warrior facing a heart transplant, he tracked down a former employee who had survived the procedure and set up a meaningful mentorship.

Human relations really kick in through this mentoring program: Think about bonding and connection based on mutual experience and common ground, or about brotherhood and a commitment to the well-being of one's peers. A level of trust and faith, born of shared suffering and affiliation, allows the wounded warrior to accept the offerings of the mentor. Once again, we see the power of community at work, with those who have been helped by others giving back to comrades whose suffering has just begun. As Scott points out, these mentors are able to make a difference:

> *The credibility is there, because if you've got a kid who is a bilateral above-the-knee amputee and he's talking to another guy who has been through the same thing, but further down the road—maybe he just competed in the wounded warrior events, or won medals in swimming and running—that does a lot to motivate him. While life is going to be different, there is still going to be a life worth living.*

Mentors are helped along in their role through education provided by 9Line. They attend seminars to learn effective communication skills, types of injuries they might encounter, and other topics that prepare them for this new line of work. Mentor meetings are held four times a year, and from Scott's perspective, they have quickly evolved into mini-reunions for the mentors and their families. "There's so much catching up to do. There is a bond with the families and different groups have formed among them. Special Operations wives, for example, meet to talk about things they're going through." These informal, spontaneous groups mirror ones that 9Line has organized proactively with structure. In fact, 9Line has created a similar group for spouses of severely injured warriors, especially those who have suffered a traumatic brain injury. The demand for this added level of support is significant since the challenges of relating to brain-injured patients are often overwhelming and all-consuming for their loved ones.

The third level of 9Line's work is the Wellness Program. This outreach operation encourages veterans to participate in activities that will improve their overall health and wellness, helping them reengage with others and with parts of themselves that may have shut down since their injury. They are introduced to organizations and community resources that will aid in their wellness goals. Scott is unabashedly enthusiastic and creative in his commitment to finding recreational outlets for his warriors: "I tell the guys if it's not illegal or immoral, ask me and we'll go from there. ... If we can find support for it, we'll try to help them. For one guy it might be fly fishing and for another it might be a triathlon."

Helping Scott in this mission is David MacDonald, another retired medevac pilot who served in operations Desert Shield and Desert Storm, as well as Operation Iraqi Freedom One. When Scott introduced Dave to 9Line's Wellness Program, he was busy starting a cattle ranch. Soon committed to the cause and to working with his mentor, Dave accepted a position with 9Line and has never looked back. His cattle ranch is fully operational, thanks to the help of a ranch foreman, and Dave is able to spend his days helping wounded warriors reclaim a critical part of their lives. Dave's perspective is this: Military personnel must maintain a high level of physical fitness in order to do what they do in the extreme situations they face every day. "When they have been wounded or injured, we show them that they can still maintain their physical fitness and their competitive spirit beyond their injury, that there are other avenues."

One especially effective and inspiring 9Line wellness project is the Wounded Warrior Athlete Program (WWAP) which partners with the United States Olympic Committee. The WWAP works with recreational athletes, some of whom become proficient enough in their sport to compete at the Olympic level. 9Line also partners with benevolent organizations around the country, offering funding for specialized equipment, training sessions, classes, and any service that will assist the wounded warrior in finding an activity or sport in which he can participate.

For athletes who want to take their sport to the next level, the WWAP will connect them with coaches and programs offered by the United States Olympic Committee through its Paralympic Military Program. The Paralympic program runs camps for a variety of sports throughout the year, where vets can assess how competitive they are, whether they want to compete, and how to get coaching if they have what it takes. Athletes are identified at the camps as being eligible for the Wounded Warrior Games, a relatively new event, now in its third year. Wounded warriors from each service branch compete against each other at the Games in a number of sports.

Supported by the Department of Defense and the U.S. Olympic Committee, the Wounded Warrior Games are a forum where the Committee can identify potential Paralympians for the international competition stage. According to Scott, "They look at the mind-set of any military guy, but especially the Special Forces, and figure the parallels are pretty tight with what a world-class athlete goes through." The Games provide a venue for all participating athletes to experience an aspect of life that had seemed unattainable since their injury. By all accounts, the Games deliver important gains of psychological wellness and connection in a population overwhelmed by feelings of isolation, loss, and marginalization.

The Wounded Warrior Games is a shining and awe-inspiring example of how sport and community can restore meaning for those who are challenged at their core. Double amputees find themselves competing on sitting volleyball teams. Those with traumatic brain injuries and severe PTSD can find comfort and solace in a safe team activity. For many, it is the first time since their injury that they have experienced the joys of sport and can take pride in their wounded bodies. In addition to the physical outlet, there is the clear psychological benefit of competing with peers on a team, with a common goal: "Like any team thing, you get benefits of being part of something, and these guys used to have that in the military, so it's a good thing to get back," reports Scott. Dave adds, "We all define ourselves as soldiers. Even those who retire like myself still miss it. You're not part of the team any more. ... You're out of the loop, and you've been doing it for so long and that's how you defined yourself." For the injured, becoming part of a team again has proven to be immensely therapeutic.

Scott and Dave both tell of a wounded warrior in their program who was battling severe depression and suicidal thoughts. He had all but given up on the possibility of a life worth living until he found himself at the 2011 Wounded Warrior Games through his involvement with 9Line. "He smiled the whole time," recalls Scott. "He's now fired up for training camp next summer." Dave adds his thoughts about the benefits of participation in the Games: "It gets them moving to set goals beyond just getting well. It helps them transition into normal life. 'I'm here, now I want to get a job.' It's a spark that ignites [their thinking about what] goal setting is all about. They need a kick start. ... I see sport as a way to do that." Once again, the experience of community turns out to be life changing and, in some cases, even lifesaving.

CrossFit is one of the organizations that has worked in conjunction with 9Line athletes and the Wounded Warrior Athlete Program with great results. Given the adaptability of the CrossFit methodology, which allows for modifications for all people and all body types, even the most severely injured athletes can improve their fitness and functionality with proper coaching and guidance. CrossFit gyms around the country open themselves up as a way for the wounded warriors to optimize their fitness and training, whatever their goals may be.

The final step in the 9Line service provision is called Reintegration. Under their contract with the Department of Defense, one of the missions of 9Line is to get as many of the wounded warriors back into operational units as possible. When this is feasible, Scott and his forces do all they can to see the mission through. However, the reality for many of the wounded in their program is that they become medically retired and need assistance finding other vocational outlets. Scott explains, "We want to be sure they get linked up with an appropriate job or get them in school or otherwise actively engaged. We don't want them sitting on the couch with a beer and a bag of chips, because obviously that leads to bad things. And then we track them. The Care Coalition, our parent unit, tracks them for life, but the advocates and mentors [also] keep in touch with them and maintain contact throughout, because they've built relationships with them and they want to make sure they're on their way."

Making sure that members of our armed forces are on their way is nothing new for Scott Heintz. Retired from the military in 2005, Scott had served twenty-six years in the United States Army as a medevac pilot, essentially taking care of soldiers throughout his career and most of his adult life. Scott's sincerity about his commitment to his work comes through loud and clear when you meet him. Humble and matter-of-fact about his mission, he is also passionate about the help he provides. Reflecting on his job as medevac pilot in the past and how it relates to his current work as head of 9Line, the depth of Scott's involvement becomes apparent:

In all of us, it's a job that you're chest deep in. You can't mail it in. It's an emotional commitment. I think that having grown up in the military and taking care of soldiers and seeing what wonderful people they are, realizing some of the challenges they're going through, I think that certainly helps. When I look to my advocates I kind of have the profile of the sergeant major, because their whole mission in life is taking care of the welfare of the kids—I say kids, I mean soldiers. They have that same commitment, that same compassion and drive to do what's right by these guys and their families. So I think all of us have that emotional background plus the skills that we obtained through hundreds of years in the military, which enable us to navigate the system and kind of call bullshit on things that are bullshit and get to a solution a little bit quicker than somebody else might be able to.

Scott was fortunate to have escaped injury throughout his service, though he surrounds himself with others who were not so lucky. He knows that engaging veterans with service disabilities is critical to 9Line's effectiveness and credibility. He talks highly of Mike Day, a former Navy SEAL and Purple Heart recipient who is now one of the 9Line Advocates and is an example of someone who can relate to the trauma many warriors have endured. Shot twenty-seven times—eleven absorbed by his vest and sixteen by his body—Mike is particularly sensitive to the needs of 9Line's clientele. "He's obviously a great advocate in terms of the perspective of having been there." Mike acknowledges the "street credibility" that his combat history and status as a severely injured veteran gives him in his new line of work. "The experiences that we went through are not something somebody else can understand. They [clients] know that I've shared maybe not the exact experience but at least something pretty damn similar. … To get on this list, you have to be classified very seriously injured, wounded or ill. It's all the worst cases." Mike even goes so far as to say that prior to getting injured he would never have been able to work with the men he now helps in the ways that are necessary:

If this didn't happen to me, there's no way I could have done this job. I was known as very unsympathetic and just a hard-nosed person. All I really wanted to do was stay in the SEAL teams and keep doing it … so if that didn't happen to me I wouldn't have been able to do this. It taught me a lot more about how to deal with other people and understanding emotions of other people. It's just what I learned when I got hurt. ... I can honestly say that I understand emotions more than I did before. ... I'm still hard-nosed, but I've learned a lot.

Dealing with the personalities of the wounded soldiers sometimes makes the work particularly challenging but also rewarding when breakthroughs occur. While some are ready to receive assistance and communicate openly about their struggles and their needs, others are more resistant and less willing to ask for help. Mike is particularly sensitive to this dynamic when dealing with veterans suffering from PTSD. He was diagnosed as having late-onset PTSD about fourteen months after he was shot repeatedly. Through his own medical treatment, he has learned that the endocrine system takes a huge hit when one's body is traumatized, so that hormonal regulation is completely "out of whack." He has found that educating his men about such factors often allows them to get the help they need: "With Special Operations guys, you're talking about all Type A personalities and to get one of them to admit that they have PTSD, which they perceive as a mental weakness, is hard to do. So if they can understand that there's physiology that they can't control that causes it to happen, then they'll go get help."

Mike's personal experiences with severe combat injuries, as well as the harrowing recovery process that follows, allows him to be especially helpful. He says, "I'm able to spot phases that they're going through in their recovery that I can recognize in my own," which leads to a greater level of empathy. Scott knows that Mike and other 9Line advocates have dealt with similar critical issues that make them well equipped to talk with the guys. "In an ideal world, all of my advocates would be folks who've been wounded but still have the skill set to navigate through the tough processes they need to get through every day." The unfortunate reality, however, is that many injured veterans suffer so much from their physical injuries and psychological trauma that they are unable to guide their cohorts through the process of reentry. Hopefully, with the work of 9Line and other support groups, this will change.

Mike has befriended every one of the guys he has helped and continues to help, and these friendships offer a unique camaraderie and connection. He has participated in the Wounded Warrior Games and plans to do so again in the future. In addition to the social connections, Mike finds perspective and grounding when he is around other wounded veterans, many of whom have far graver injuries than his, serious as they were: "It helps me to be around those guys. When you're around a bunch of people who are amputees and worse than that—guys that have been shot in the head. ... If they're out there, it kind of makes it easier for you to do it. It's kind of hard to complain about anything when you're around those people." Mike especially enjoys arranging "wellness trips" when wounded warriors spend time together participating in an activity. These opportunities for socializing and engaging in something physical in the outdoors "help an awful lot," according to Mike.

We have seen that the human connections at the core of the military community are strong and lasting. Scott explains how shared suffering and experience in the trenches does, indeed, lead to a unique level of connectedness:

There's a brotherhood. Within each service there are subgroups where that bond is even tighter. I was one of the medevac guys and still have a circle of one hundred and fifty to two hundred people interconnected. I still talk to lots of them often. The Special Operations community—because of the nature of dangerous missions and the fact that they are deployed remotely in austere environments in small teams—they become very close. Then sub that group out again with those that are wounded, and that's an even tighter brotherhood. Then you give them something like the Wounded Warrior Games or this program. Most of these guys didn't know each other. At the Wounded Warrior Games they just bonded throughout. There was a lot of talk of "Wait till next year. We're going to do this for training, etcetera." The shared experience of going to war, of being wounded, of being put in dangerous situations, creates a bond among these guys that you don't find in other professions.

Mike echoes Scott's sentiments: "We all stay in touch. These guys know, they can tell by the way I help them out ... that I'm not just doing this because it's a paycheck. I mean they literally are all my friends."

Operation Phoenix: Jimi Letchford and CrossFit in Support of Our Troops

By all accounts, CrossFit founder Greg Glassman has always had an eye on helping our troops develop and maintain fitness levels to optimize their ability to perform and stay safe while doing their important work. Early in the creation of CrossFit, Glassman had already started reaching out to military personnel, spreading the word about how CrossFit could be used as a training program to prepare for the rigors of combat. In 2007, when it was time to close the doors at CrossFit Santa Cruz—the first CrossFit gym where it had all begun—Glassman donated all of the equipment to the Marines at Camp Pendleton. Operation Phoenix was the name given to the delivery, transport, and installation of the Santa Cruz gym gear, worth more than $60,000.

When Jimi Letchford was seven years old, his father, a police officer in southern New Jersey, took him to a father-son wrestling camp at the United States Naval Academy in Annapolis, Maryland. Jimi had been to many other camps in his early years, but there was something special about this one. Jimi was awestruck by the Naval Academy and decided he wanted to end up at a place where there's a jet outside your classroom. As he got older, he learned more about the Naval Academy and the education he could get there, and it became more than just a cool place with big jets. He remembers thinking, "This is a great deal. I can go to college and get a killer degree. I can have a job on the way out, and I can serve my country and do some really neat things. So I went to the Academy with all that intent, just wanting to be where the rubber hits the road."

Timing is everything. Jimi was at the Academy on September 11, 2001. Along with his comrades throughout our military, Jimi went from training for the future to immediate preparations for combat. When he graduated in 2003, Jimi was commissioned as a marine officer, promoted to first commander in 2004, and deployed twice to Iraq over the next two years.

Jimi's entry into the United States Marine Corps was a positive, conscious choice. At some point during his education, Jimi had heard a briefing about a marine back in the 1990s who was part of a training operation practicing transport of marines onto a ship. The training mission went awry when a CH46 helicopter went over, clipping a cable on the ship and rolling into the water. The platoon commander and a couple of others survived, but several marines did not. Following the tragic accident, Jimi recalls hearing about the fund-raising efforts of a fellow marine: "This marine had been running Ironmans and triathlons and all kinds of crazy races, and he had been winning them all so that he could raise money for their children, for their educations. I was like, 'That's the kind of guy I want to serve with. I want to serve with that kind of brotherhood.' So I decided to go into the Marine Corps."

A competitive wrestler in college, Jimi was always searching for a fitness program that would satisfy his training needs and feed his competitive drives after graduation. Though he tried mixed martial arts and triathlons, he wasn't satisfied. When one of his marines approached him with great enthusiasm about a fitness program he had found on the Internet called CrossFit, Jimi gave it a try and was hooked. He followed the workouts and instruction on CrossFit.com for a couple of years on his own and with some of his Marine Corps buddies.

Jimi became a Marine Corps commander at the School of Infantry, where trainees are readied for battle. Part of his job was to supervise the training of soldiers coming straight out of boot camp. "Our job was to train them to shoot, move, and communicate before they went off on their deployment. We had eight weeks of instruction to get these guys ready. ... They'd come in fit to run, do pull-ups, stuff like that, but they weren't used to the type of training it takes to become a marine." Injuries were common and dropout rates were high, due to a lack of preparedness for the rigors of training. Then something changed: In 2006, Jimi was given the opportunity to attend a CrossFit certification in Canada. He spent three days learning from some of the best coaches CrossFit had to offer, including Glassman himself, all with an eye on how CrossFit might be worked into training for the Marines. "I was blown away. I thought it was amazing. It was exactly what I ... thought marines needed, especially on the front lines—training for the unknown and unknowable. I was super excited about what I had learned and how it could apply to our guys."

Every two weeks, 200 to 400 marines would start at the School of Infantry in a new company. They woke up early, worked hard, and ran through a full range of physical activities before meeting with Jimi for fitness training that was supplemental to their already demanding regimen. Jimi did the CrossFit programming himself, since there were unique challenges of implementation with a group of 300 guys working out at the same time. In true CrossFit style, he and his team improvised: "We did sprints, hauled sandbags, ammo cans, we got our hands on some old truck tires you could flip and jump on. We did buddy carries out on the range." At first, there was some resistance to the training; it was challenging and the marines were tired. But soon, the feedback was loud and clear: more CrossFit. Jimi and the other officers noticed immediate results. Based on pre- and post-fitness testing, they saw thirty percent gains in overall scores. More surprisingly, though, they also noticed huge improvements in the academic performance of the trainees and far fewer injuries. Whereas they had previously averaged fifteen to forty-five recruits who were "rolled back" because of injury, they now made it through two full classes without a single injury. Clearly, the program was working, and Jimi was ecstatic.

Over time, Jimi maintained contact with Coach Glassman via email, mostly checking in to let him know how well the program was working for his troops. At some point, Glassman invited Jimi to be part of the CrossFit Headquarters training team, giving him the opportunity to travel around the world and help at training seminars like the one he had attended in Canada. Jimi was present when Operation Phoenix went down, and he remembers Glassman's fervent commitment to providing that kind of equipment delivery for every military and first responder unit in the country. The idea was big, the goal was lofty, but the motivation was there, and these were CrossFitters. Glassman asked Jimi to spearhead the continuation of Operation Phoenix which would involve raising funds by selling T-shirts, with 100 percent of the profits going toward equipment purchases for, and deliveries to, military bases. They started with the Marine Corps, but the goal was to branch out to all the armed services and first responder units in the country—providing for anyone whose life depended upon his or her strength and fitness.

Along the way, Operation Phoenix was stalled by red tape. Certain government-contracted companies were not pleased about having free equipment delivery and free fitness training provided to the military; the military was their customer and free training threatened their profitability. Since that time, however, the CrossFit Foundation has received authorization for the equipment drops, and Operation Phoenix is up and running and is about to take on a whole new level of service. Under Jimi's direction and in partnership with Rogue Fitness, the largest manufacturer of CrossFit equipment, Operation Phoenix will now have a gift registry through which military and first responder units will be able to get exactly what they need for their fitness training. Each unit will go through an authentication process and, once approved, will create a registry requesting the gear they need. This way people in the CrossFit community or supporters of our troops and first responders—anyone, really—will be able to purchase exactly what is needed at each base or unit. Jimi is excited about how this registry will help outfit those in need, and he likes the idea that "it puts the onus on the units to take accountability for their own registry and their own support." Also, as he points out, this system will allow unit commanders whose fitness equipment needs are well funded to help out other units lacking the same resources, thereby tapping into community support from within.

Asked about the philanthropic nature of the CrossFit community and why so many people are driven to help others, Jimi has this to say:

Everyone recognizes that we are part of something huge. This community is big, and it's full of people who care. They care about themselves. They care about each other. They care about community. You wouldn't be doing CrossFit if you didn't care about yourself on some level. It's hard. If it were easy, everyone would be doing it, because it works. So that's one level. You come to know the people in the community, whether virtually following the online workouts on CrossFit.com or in person [at a gym]. They come for the community. I think we all recognize that we have the ability to affect something. Whether it's a local thing or a local family or something national or something we want to bring attention to. It's a lifestyle. Lifestyle's not just about what kind of car you drive, what kind of clothes you wear, or what you do on your vacation. Lifestyle is this mind-

set, it's this overarching Chi. It's "You know what, I'm fit, I feel good, I'm happy." I'm here to help people and make the community better. Not just our community, but everybody—a paying it forward type of thing.

This all could sound idealistic and even corny if it weren't so simple and real. To be part of it firsthand, to know that you can call on a group of people and raise $15,000 in a matter of days in support of a cause is truly inspiring. In our own TJ's Gym community, we've done it for breast cancer, for a local child with cancer whose medical bills had piled up, for families of fallen soldiers, and for inner-city kids. We've seen the positive psychological energy created when individuals come together for their workouts with a common goal. Success is fueled by an appreciation of the will, effort, and reward of doing something difficult and meaningful, and doing it with others. Another element involves the respect and empathy for what someone else is going through because you may have experienced it yourself.

In exploring the parallels between military and CrossFit efforts, Jimi notes,

[Being in the military] is tough. It's tough on a family and it's tough on the individuals, but that builds ... camaraderie between the guys and the girls that you serve next to, because they're going through the same thing. There are different calibers, different levels, but you're spending a lot of time with people, and you trust them for a number of reasons. Their family is your family's support network back home, and they are your support network going forward. ... I think that's similar to what we're seeing in the CrossFit community right now. ... You go into any box or training with any friends and that shared suffering is something that really pulls people together. It's the workouts when you're in the gym, people are going hard and you know what that person is going through.

... If you finish before them, you're turning around and you know what they're feeling right at that moment because you were just there. ... It builds this bond between you that is almost inseparable.

It is from these connections that communities are built and resources are shared. Operation Phoenix is another stellar example of how the CrossFit Foundation (crossfitfoundation.com) spreads its wealth of funds, spirit, and assistance.

Bo's Story

Bo Dahlberg was twenty years old in July of 2005 when he joined the United States Coast Guard Reserves, the premier maritime law enforcement service. Bo chose this path in order to gain experience that would bring him closer to his long-term goal of becoming a police officer.

Bo's father worked for the San Francisco Police Department for more than twenty-five years. As a child and adolescent, Bo was fascinated by his father's work, and he often accompanied his dad on his beat in the city. Bo was especially struck by the respectful way his father dealt with the diversity of people he encountered every day, "from the big shots who owned the high rises, to the florist lady, to the homeless man lying on the sidewalk." He was also impressed by the respect his father received in return. Bo filled his free time learning about military equipment, reading extensively and perusing pictures in the Encyclopedia of the Military.

In high school, his interest in the military intensified, and he participated in his high school's Army JROTC program. He liked its focus on creating future citizens through discipline. He believed in the importance of the character traits necessary for military service—honor, respect, courage, and commitment to duty—all instilled in him and his cohorts during their time in the JROTC.

Bo studied administration of justice in junior college, preparing him for a future in law enforcement. All the while, he was employed in physically demanding jobs, making enough money to support himself and spending time outside, which suited him far more than studying indoors. When Bo was old enough to become a police officer, he chose the Coast Guard as a stepping stone to that law enforcement career and a way to pursue the ideals of his JROTC training:

I knew I had to do something honorable to show my level of commitment and maturity, so I enlisted. It wasn't a big deal to me. I always wanted to enlist, and to this day, I still could make a career out of it. By enlisting in the military and having a deployment under my belt, I had a "leg up" on other applicants my age. College is great and all, but the most important skill to have in law enforcement is common sense.

Bo's career in the Coast Guard has provided him with several years of challenge and elite training that would serve him well in the future. He reflects on his early time in the Coast Guard, describing his experiences during his two deployments overseas:

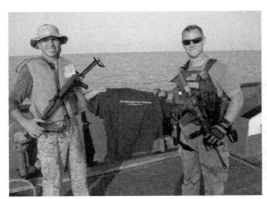 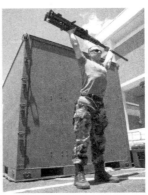

Bo Dahlberg (right) while deployed in the North Arabian Gulf and living on the Al Basarah Oil Terminal and working with a member of the Iraqi Marines (left).

Bo at Air Station San Francisco with an M2 .50 machine gun.

After basic training, I was attached to Port Security Unit 312, an expeditionary unit whose primary mission was to provide force protection, antiterrorism, and law enforcement capabilities to high-value assets around the world. We wear camouflage uniforms, Kevlar helmets, body armor, and deploy with other branches of service around the world. When people think of the USCG, they think of the orange helicopters, big white ships, and dudes jumping out of helicopters saving people. So I guess that made us the bastard step-child of the Coast Guard—the way we liked it.

I attended the Maritime Enforcement Specialist "A" School (formerly, Port Security Specialist School) in Yorktown, Virginia. We were taught defensive tactics (handcuffing, control holds, take-downs, etc.), maritime laws, weapon handling, vessel-boarding techniques. It was a good start for my future career in law enforcement. I found out I thrived in a military environment. I loved the training, the stress, and the teamwork. I later found out I really liked the lifestyle as well. Wake up, do some PT (physical training), go to work, do some more PT, go to bed, wake up and do it again. Very regimented, but I enjoyed it. I graduated as the Honor-Man at the top of my class.

In addition to various training evolutions around the San Francisco Bay Area and the country, I was deployed twice during my six years with the Coast Guard, first to Guantanamo Bay, Cuba, where I served as a tactical boat crewman. We provided waterside security for the naval base, as well as security for any detainee movement operation.

I was also deployed to the Middle East for eight months. I started working in Kuwait at the Al Shuwaba Sea Port of Deportation (SPOD). This is where all equipment going to and from Iraq and Afghanistan traveled. At any point in time there were millions of dollars of military assets on the ground, from Humvees to tanks to Blackhawk helicopters. We worked alongside our Army counterparts and were stationed at numerous Entry Control Points (ECPs). Throughout the deployment we searched thousands of vehicles and personnel and provided security for SPOD.

While the majority of my unit was dedicated to that mission, I did most of my deployment on the A Basrah Oil Platform (ABOT). There I was the Special Response Team leader, responsible for internal platform defense and boarding and searching any vessels that were transiting to the platform. We also worked alongside the British Royal Marine Commandos and other Coast Guard personnel training the Iraqi Marines in Close Quarters Combat and maritime interdiction operations. My team and I conducted over sixty vessel boardings, responded to multiple medical emergencies on the platform, and completed many training evolutions. It was stressful some of the time and hot all the time. On the platform, we worked alongside the Iraqi Marines and provided platform defense. ABOT was responsible for over ninety percent of Iraq's revenue and was considered one of the top ten terrorist targets in the world. Although I never saw combat, I conducted "higher"-risk boardings and was involved in strategic situations on the platform.

I completed my contract with the Coast Guard in July of 2011 as a Maritime Enforcement Specialist 2nd Class, a rank equivalent to an Army Sergeant. Another major accomplishment during my enlistment was being selected to attend and complete the U.S. Marine Corps Urban Leaders Course. This rigorous, competitive, month-long course at Camp Pendleton, California, covered urban combat, also known as MOUT (military operations, urban terrain) or Close Quarter Battle (CQB). We trained alongside the Marines, conducting training missions using Simunitions (a soap-based projectile fired out of a real weapon, accurate and hurts like hell, a great training tool). We learned convoy operations, IED characteristics, participated in numerous live-fire training exercises with various weapons systems including the AK-47. Also covered in great detail was the "warrior" or "combat" mind-set—what physically and mentally happens to your body during a gun fight and what to be aware of. Every morning we PT'd [physical trained] from carrying a "wounded" comrade over a mile to an extraction area, to running over three miles in full gear with resupplies. My favorite workout was a two-mile run with a mouthful of water.

Not surprisingly, Bo has experienced a strong sense of community during his service in the Coast Guard. Having worked with so many different branches of the military, he has a unique perspective of the community as a whole. He is quick to point out that the military is comprised of people from all walks of life, with different backgrounds, goals, and philosophies. Despite this, bonding occurs because they have all made a significant sacrifice: "Everyone (in the military) has been in an uncomfortable and unknown situation at some time. … Everyone has been away from their families. Everyone has felt sad, homesick. But everyone has also felt alive. So there is that unspoken rule of respect and consideration for one another." That bond intensifies with comrades in service, as Bo explains:

I compare it to that special friend that everyone has. The one where life gets busy and you don't talk to that person in months, then all of a sudden you meet up and everything is back where it left off. I compare my relationships with my brothers and sisters in arms to that. We've all seen each other in uncomfortable situations, in varying degrees of sadness and joy. Sat alongside them when they found out they are a father to a new baby boy. The great thing in the military is the camaraderie. It is a simple life where you live in the moment. Whether you had a stressful encounter, did not receive any mail, or saw your best friend die. A life where people reflect on their experiences all the time.

In October 2007, while still part of the USCG, Bo enrolled in the 140th Alameda County Sheriff's Office Basic Law Enforcement Academy, known for its high academic standards and demanding physical testing. This, Bo says, is where "I found my niche in physical fitness. Having a strong mind and not showing any pain worked well for me. I enjoyed being given a physically demanding task and throwing myself at it." It was after graduating from the Academy and joining the Alamada County Sheriff's Office that Bo found TJ's Gym and discovered CrossFit: "I was searching for something like an academy. Something challenging. Something different every day. Something I could throw myself at. I still could practice my war face, because other gym members were around. I walked through the doors … and fell in love."

Bo's Coast Guard service parallels his involvement with CrossFit and the TJ's Gym crew. He points to the "family atmosphere … the people, the community, being around people who push themselves to that dark place, all in the name of becoming a better citizen, a better human on this Earth. Who wouldn't want to surround themselves with people like that?" Bo finds common ground between his comrades in the military and his workout buddies at TJ's Gym:

People join the military to better themselves, to provide service to their country. When they leave they have the skills, confidence, and experience to help them succeed in the world. At TJ's it's the same thing. People come from all walks of life to better themselves, to provide a small yet important service to their community. They are able-bodied, strong-willed, confident individuals. Through experiences and workouts, they have the know-how to focus on that all-important acronym: WIN—What's Important Now? TJ's and the military put everything into focus. Whether it's just to get a good workout or to conquer their weak minds, people become better human beings through difficult and demanding situations.

Indeed, when Bo found himself in difficult and demanding situations during deployment, the internalized self-confidence and determination he had cultivated through CrossFit workouts grounded him and kept him calm:

Through my experiences training at TJ's, my body developed a better understanding of pain and discomfort. I had a better sense of what my body was capable of and how far I could push it. This gave me a huge boost in confidence—whether it was climbing on an old disintegrating tire to board a dhow (Iraqi fishing vessel), to walking alongside a general, in full armor, helmet, and weapons, providing personal protection while he toured an Iraqi oil platform with the heat index at 140 degrees. I remembered all those tough WODs where I thought I couldn't finish, but did. And sometimes, to my surprise, I did remarkably well. So I wiped the sweat from my eyes, tightened up my core, ignored all the symptoms of heat cramps, and pushed through.

It wasn't just the physical results of his workouts that propelled Bo. He also made a lasting relationship while deployed in Kuwait through the camaraderie of CrossFit training. Bo and his buddy, Justin, a Royal Marine Commando from southern England, managed to rig a gym on their platform in Kuwait since many of the CrossFit movements were not permitted in the base gym—the workouts required too much space or involved the dropping of weights as in a deadlift, which was apparently not allowed. "Our gym on the platform was in between two heated forty-eight-inch oil pipes mixed up with more pipes and old spilled oil. Some dirty camouflage netting provided shade and a dilapidated railing kept us from falling off the platform into the sea some forty feet below. But it was awesome! Everything was rusty, but we made do with what we had. Being deployed is a lot like being a kid again. You get dirty, you get yourself into some stupid situations, and everyone tries to make the best of nothing." Bo and Justin still correspond to this day, updating each other on their fitness progress as well as other aspects of their lives.

Bo is currently still technically in the USCG, a member of the inactive ready reserve (IRR) for the next two years. He states, "Unless WWIII breaks out, I'm good." He is now deputy sheriff with the Marin County Sheriff's Office, a job he loves, in part because of its variety: "I go from Section Eight housing to million-dollar homes in about 120 seconds, depending on how fast I drive. From people on welfare who sell drugs and have guns shoved in their waistbands, to the rich hoity-toity, "I pay your salary" or "You are MY public servant!" ... and everywhere in between. That's why I love the County."

Bo plans to use this time in his life to focus on his career with the Sheriff's Office, spend time with his wife and family, and dedicate himself to working out at TJ's Gym. Reflecting on the importance of his workouts and the connections he has made, Bo states:

I feel that CrossFit and TJ's Gym will some day save my life. Each workout I participate in is my fight for survival. I try to look strong at all times, to save face, and take something away from each workout. Just like my experiences in the military, CrossFit provides me with daily "uncomforts" in a world full of comforts. To realize that life isn't only about going to work, making money, and going home. It's a time where it doesn't matter what's going on later in the day. A time to be loud, to be aggressive, and to come out on top. ... It's a chance to feel alive and live it up a bit, to enjoy the camaraderie of getting fit.

Chapter 9

The Corporate Community: The Reebok/CrossFit Initiative

In September 2010, CrossFit Incorporated and Reebok International joined forces in a partnership that would link Reebok to the CrossFit Games for years to come. The hallmark of the agreement is Reebok's sponsorship of the Games, which included a million-dollar prize purse for athletes at the competition for the fittest in the world at the 2011 Games, as well as a wardrobe overhaul for all participating athletes.

When news of Reebok's involvement with CrossFit first surfaced in 2010, there was quite a bit of skepticism among CrossFitters worldwide. Because CrossFit began as a grassroots movement purposefully free of corporate sponsorship, it has a following of purists. Fears emerged that the big corporate Goliath might dictate how affiliate owners could run their gyms or put them out of business by opening mega-Reebok/CrossFit gyms on every street corner.

People wondered if the Reebok executives would understand the culture of CrossFit and the importance of the existing community and customs. There was much talk about Greg Glassman selling out and risking the integrity of the CrossFit movement by merging with a corporate giant.

Glassman explained that the association with Reebok was born of a mutual understanding of the needs and desires of CrossFit affiliate owners and athletes worldwide. He spoke about the sincerity of the motivations of the folks at Reebok—how they appreciated the essence of CrossFit and would not threaten the heart and soul of the operation. He talked about how the Reebok people could help further the mission of CrossFit to promote its fitness philosophy. They would allow the CrossFit Games to be grander and more exciting than ever before, and there was nothing bad about that. Indeed, the million-dollar purse was sure to be a welcomed addition, as would the ability to introduce events that might otherwise not be feasible. Time would tell if the CrossFit community would accept the merger and the 2011 CrossFit Games was, for some, as much a proving ground of corporate involvement as it was for finding the fittest in the world.

As an athlete and affiliate team member representing TJ's Gym/ CrossFit San Rafael, I had an insider's view of the Reebok-sponsored Games. Within hours of arriving at the hotel in Carson, California, we were greeted by a team from Reebok who outfitted our team with a full selection of customized workout clothes and accessories, making us feel like professional athletes. There was even a tailor on hand for immediate alterations! While the quantity of gear was overwhelming, what was most noteworthy was how focused the Reebok people were on augmenting our experience and meeting our needs as athletes. From the staff unpacking boxes and delivering our uniforms, to the designers who asked us for feedback on style and function over the course of the weekend, the entire crew was attentive and impressive. The executives were also involved throughout, approachable and willing to chat about the motivation behind partnering with CrossFit, handing out business cards for follow-up, requesting our ideas about how Reebok could be helpful to CrossFit gym owners and athletes alike.

I have since spoken with many Reebok employees and executives who have been open and forthcoming about their affiliation with CrossFit. They acknowledge the benefits and rewards of the process of integrating into the larger CrossFit community. Beyond the excitement of having been introduced to a new and dynamic fitness regimen, the Reebok people have been touched by the camaraderie and connections made during workouts, inspired by the emotional and relational benefits of their involvement with CrossFit. While the Reebok/CrossFit relationship is still a work in progress, and partnerships of this magnitude can change course with time, the foundation appears to be built on shared goals and mutual understanding. That being said, Reebok is a corporation invested in the bottom line, with a goal to expand and promote its brand. It is not just in this out of the goodness of its corporate heart. We may see more Reebok-sponsored CrossFit gyms appearing around the world in the near future. This collaboration can be a positive force as long as the new gyms respect the existing affiliate structure and further the CrossFit goals of excellence in fitness and human potential.

Improving the Lives of Employees

Corporations often have missions that guide their acquisitions, marketing, customer relations, and overall operations. These missions change from time to time, which is why companies sometimes change direction. In early 2010, Reebok had declared its mission to become the premier fitness and training brand within the next five years. According to Head of Human Resources, Bill Holmes, Reebok wanted consumers to come to identify Reebok as *the* fitness brand. The Reebok/CrossFit initiative was one measure implemented to reach this goal. In addition to partnering with CrossFit at the

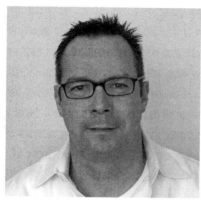

Bill Holmes, Head of Human Resources, Reebok International.

sponsorship level, the executives at Reebok were driven to create a culture of fitness within the corporation itself. While Reebok had always encouraged its employees to be fit and active, there was now a new intensity, focus, and structure to that encouragement. Sparked by their relationship with CrossFit, Reebok created a program called "3, 2, 1 … Go!" These are the words most CrossFitters hear from their coaches just prior to starting the clock on their workouts. These words would now encompass an entire health and wellness initiative for the employees of Reebok worldwide.

In May 2011, all Reebok employees in Canton received an email jointly sent from Bill Holmes, Head of Human Resources, Uli Becker, Brand President, and Matt O'Toole, Chief Marketing Officer. Carefully crafted to strongly urge company-wide attendance, the email explained that there would be a workout on the lawn outside the offices on May 18. According to Holmes, the email read: "You are expected to attend." The executives hoped that every last employee would show up but were acutely aware of the reputation CrossFit had around campus. Among those who weren't yet hooked, the word on the street was that CrossFit was scary, intense, and especially hardcore. Apparently the email worked, as well over 700 employees gathered on the lawn that day and participated in an introductory

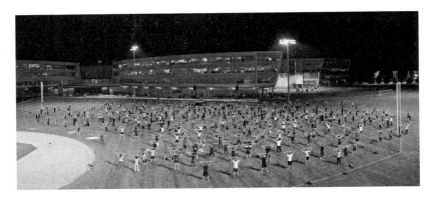

CrossFit Experience workout at Reebok International Headquarters, May, 2011.

community workout led by some of New England's finest CrossFit coaches. Holmes attributes much of what has transpired since then to the success and power of that first group workout: "That event was the catalyst for the culture of fitness at Reebok."

Bryant Mitchell, Affiliate Relationship Manager at Reebok, recalls being "blown away" by that workout on the lawn. Having spent years in the corporate fitness world selling fitness health and wellness programs to companies, Bryant came to Reebok in May of 2011. One of his first experiences was the group workout, and he was immediately impressed by the support of Reebok executives for CrossFit as the main component of its fitness initiative. Crucial for Bryant was that the support was so clearly genuine, a result of personal experiences with the effectiveness of the workouts and the meaningful relationships they had helped develop:

I had never seen a company embrace and encourage physical fitness and activity the way that Reebok had. And ... my background is corporate fitness and wellness. I was acting as a consultant helping businesses pursue a corporate fitness and wellness strategy. We always knew the key driver was support from the top down. If you have your key executives encouraging participation, it's going to be more successful. If they don't, then you'll struggle. ... Well 700 people went through a CrossFit workout that day at Reebok. We called it the CrossFit Experience. ... Our CEO was on stage talking about what CrossFit meant for him, what it had done for him, and then Matt O'Toole, Chief Marketing Officer, gets on stage and talks about what it's meant for him and done for him personally. And then Chris Froio, Head of Fitness and Training, gets on stage and talks about it. It really just blew me away. There were people who had been CrossFitting, but many more who had never tried it. Then we go out and do a 700-person workout and it's fun and everything is scaled and everyone is doing some version of the same movement. ... My initial observation was wow, talk about support from the top down. ... Everybody who was anybody was out there.

Prior to that 700-person workout, many Reebok employees had already been benefiting from the introduction of the CrossFit program at Reebok months before. Indeed, Reebok One, the name of the CrossFit gym at corporate headquarters, was by then preparing to field a team of athletes who would compete at the CrossFit Northeast Regionals. Hundreds of employees had already noticed gains in their energy levels, made changes in their ways of eating for optimal health and wellness, and had lost extra pounds put on over the years. In addition to these measurable results, something else was happening. A community was emerging from within the walls of the "box," a nickname for CrossFit gyms that took hold at Reebok and is now what the most enthusiastic of the employee CrossFitters call their home away from home.

A business decision to sponsor a fitness competition has deeply affected the daily lives and long-term wellness of large numbers of employees of Reebok International. Who could have predicted that this partnership would propel hundreds of individuals in offices at

Reebok headquarters to commit to working out together and sharing nutritional goals? Who could have imagined that the water cooler conversation would focus on how the workout went that morning and what might be achieved next time? The change has been positive and remarkable. In a matter of months a corporate culture has shifted, and employee relations have been enriched and strengthened. While Glassman and the Reebok heads of state hoped for this type of corporate overhaul, my sense from talking to a number of people closely involved is that the scope and impact of Reebok's partnership with CrossFit has surprised just about everyone.

So far the merger appears to be going exceedingly well, with CrossFitters around the world becoming more and more convinced that Reebok's intentions derive from an authentic passion for the CrossFit program. While the idea is to make money and expand marketing opportunities, the people involved at Reebok CrossFit genuinely get what the movement is all about and appear to be invested in furthering the characteristics of CrossFit that have made it special. The Reebok

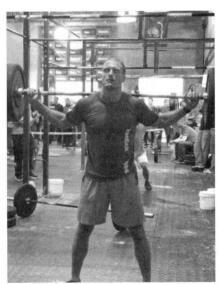

Bryant Mitchell, Manager, Affiliate & Community Services, Reebok International. Member of Reebok One.

professionals understand that the most compelling, influential, and powerful aspect of CrossFit may well be the community it creates, and by choosing CrossFit, they are on to something much bigger than just a fun and effective workout.

One of Reebok's goals in creating a community of fitness was to foster the relationship between male and female coworkers. Both Bill and Bryant independently highlighted this area of corporate culture. Bryant has noticed a marked difference between the company in Canton and the companies where he had worked in the past. In prior corporate settings, the default was a kind of "boys club" in which male workers would do things together outside of work, bonding in ways that gave them relationships exclusive of the women in the company. Bryant acknowledges that "it just happened" that way. Part of the boys club atmosphere included playing sports such as golf and squash in which women did not participate. However, at Reebok, Bryant and others now enjoy the opportunity to exercise together with both men and women. "CrossFit is for everybody. There's an opportunity for women who may not have had the chance to sweat with a coworker in a co-ed environment—an opportunity to work out with men."

Reebok has always had a strong female presence and has historically been a fitness brand embraced by women (remember the 1980s aerobics scene in America?). While the corporate culture has reflected this, there has been a remarkable and noticeable cultural shift along gender lines since the arrival of CrossFit on campus, according to Bill, who has been at Reebok for almost twenty years:

In a CrossFit Box the equality of what goes on in that community is very powerful. ... Our workouts and our participation prior to CrossFit was way more solitary, way more individualistic. While we may have had basketball games or softball games or various flag football pickup games, the community of men and women working out together had

*never remotely been as strong as it is today. ... Women have
always worked out ... and have always been well respected
and represented when it comes to fitness [at Reebok], but I
don't think they've participated shoulder to shoulder the way
that they do in the CrossFit Box. It's one of the most amazing
communities that I've ever witnessed ... and I've played sports
all my life.*

The even playing field provided by CrossFit has led to some of
my favorite moments as a CrossFit affiliate owner. In a community
where moms of young children reclaiming their pre-baby bodies and
fitness levels work out alongside twenty-something men who are
reclaiming their glory days from the high school or college football
field, moments of surprise and special joy abound. The mom in her
late thirties with ninety-five pounds on her barbell every so often
moves more quickly and effortlessly than the football player, and the
accompanying emotions and reactions are priceless.

Furthering the concept of the even playing field, Bryant points
out that the CrossFit experience at Reebok has brought together
executives and lower-level employees in ways he has never seen
in other companies. The increased access to business leaders is a
significant benefit to the corporate culture as a whole. Working out
alongside your boss, sharing moments of struggle and perseverance,
cheering each other on during times of physical challenge, provides
for a unique sense of connection and equality. Both Bryant and Bill
agree that it is not just the relationship between the executives and the
employees that has evolved since the introduction of CrossFit. There
is generally a renewed sense of closeness and camaraderie among all
company employees, based on a mutual understanding of the effort,
self-reflection, commitment, and lifestyle changes the demanding
workouts and overall fitness program require.

Bill enthusiastically describes the changes he has witnessed:

Brand new friendships are being born. More people are getting to know each other through CrossFit and through this fitness culture than would have ever known each other before. ... It's done a lot for the respect level of people for senior management and senior management for all employees, because we're working out side by side, we're participating. ... It's definitely having a profound effect ... cross-functionally, where people who may never have interacted together because of their different departments are now working out together. I hear through and through that people respect that [the senior managers are doing it]. It's the credibility that comes along with the new relationships, the new partnerships. "Hey that's who so and so is," and "Hey, have you met this person?" It's started a fire in the organization, and it's burning in a very positive way.

As a CrossFitter prior to the Reebok/CrossFit partnership, Chief Marketing Officer, Matt O'Toole, had been struck by the social and communal aspects of working out at CrossFit New England. He describes the whole CrossFit experience as "a community-based way to stay connected to your own personal goals but also be part of something bigger." Matt has also noticed the changes in the community feel at Reebok, an especially rewarding outcome for him. Indeed, the drive for community in exercise was a large part of what had motivated him to connect with Greg Glassman and to spearhead the Reebok-CrossFit initiative in the first place.

Matt, Bill, and Bryant agree that the overall fitness culture at Reebok has been fueled by CrossFit. For Bill, who was a driving force behind the "3, 2, 1" program and stands behind the fitness initiative at Reebok, the all-inclusive nature of the general fitness offerings are critical to the success of the initiative. He notes that part of his role is to encourage employees to just move, by walking, running, or going to the traditional Reebok gym. An employee incentive program for walking a certain number of miles over a designated period of time is but one example of a program Bill and his personnel are pushing. The point is to involve as many employees in the health and wellness movement as possible, and while one of the goals is admittedly to get as many of them doing CrossFit as possible, steps along the way are considered meaningful and legitimate gains. So far, Bill has been quite pleased with Reebok's "conversion rates," by which he means the numbers of workers who have turned to CrossFit for their exercise program.

A big issue for human resource professionals is the level of productivity of the workforce. The idea is to have happy and healthy employees who are more motivated, more driven, and more energized as they approach their jobs. Research has demonstrated the positive connection between healthy employees and productivity, a factor not lost on employers, especially those whose global mission is to become a fitness brand.[39] The data shows that preventive fitness programs, though costly in the short-term, can greatly reduce long-term expenditures related to employee healthcare.[40]

Asked about this cost-benefit analysis and whether Reebok has any hard statistics to support the positive effects of its fitness initiative, Bill Holmes is convinced that something unique and positive is happening. He talks about the increase in employee engagement, productivity and spirit. He explains how Reebok's attractiveness to job seekers has improved dramatically. He notes that managers are encouraged to "cajole" employees to do something active and to take the time to work out effectively, while making it clear that "this culture is not an excuse to miss a deadline or underperform." Holmes remarks: "I have not seen the energy, positive attitude, the spirit this good in a long, long time. ... It's created a very genuine new energy in the building. ... We like what we see. That's probably good enough data right now." There is far more to it than crunching numbers, and Bill clearly understands this:

We have good employees and good human beings ... who work here at Reebok. When you take them and bring them together in a community, in this case we'll call it CrossFit, ... magic happens. ... We've given them a Northern Light, a purpose, a direction. ... We [senior managers] also know in our hearts what we're doing is good and right and appropriate for our employees. We're trying to help people. We have a phrase here: We're trying to empower people to be fit for life. And that's an honorable cause, so when we do these events and when we have these initiatives ... we know that our intentions are very genuine and very true, and that gives me a pretty clear conscience.

Echoing these sentiments, Matt describes employees as being "much more lit up and energized about their work" and "more proud of their company" for the progressive changes at Reebok, including healthier food options in the cafeteria and offerings for sponsorship at CrossFit Level One certifications so that employees can educate themselves about health and wellness.

Bryant Mitchell is equally passionate about the positive impact that the Reebok/CrossFit partnership has had in creating a working community within the organization:

The fitness industry has been looking for the magic pill for years. And the magic pill is camaraderie and creating an experience that transcends the actual workout or WOD [workout of the day]. It's much more than the physical. And that makes it THE most effective application for the corporate environment. ... It's just amazing.

The fact that many of Bryant's coworkers need new pants because their waistlines have shrunk or that many of Bill's subordinates are carrying different foods in their lunch bags is a testament to the effectiveness of CrossFit as a physical fitness program. However, there is something even more significant at work psychologically, emotionally, and relationally, and this is what will drive the sustainability of the "3, 2,1" program as Reebok moves forward with its CrossFit partnership. Given the known benefits of community, it is not surprising that human connections transcend the workouts, and nurturing these connections within the walls of the CrossFit gym gives the program its unique power. The following story will illuminate the process of change that is taking place at Reebok.

Peggy Baker
It's Never Too Late

Peggy Baker was always overweight as a kid. She shopped in the "chubby" clothes section of department stores. Her mom was overweight. Her father was thin but sedentary. Encouraged by her mother, who didn't want to see Peggy follow in her footsteps, Peggy tried Weight Watchers and various other exercise and nutrition programs over the years, with little to no success. When Peggy turned thirty and became pregnant, she was diagnosed with gestational diabetes and was one of the unlucky women for whom the condition continued after pregnancy. She was diagnosed with Type 2 diabetes and was immediately prescribed insulin therapy. Doctors urged Peggy to make lifestyle changes, but even with her diagnosis spurring her on, she had a hard time making any lasting changes and was weighed down by an attitude of "I can't do that."

Peggy works in the IT department at Reebok, where she has been for more than twenty-seven years. Initially doing data entry and later switchboard work, she now heads up wireless for the North American region. Peggy is amused and amazed that she has experienced all of her major life events as a Reebok employee: "I got married here, divorced here, married here, had a child here."

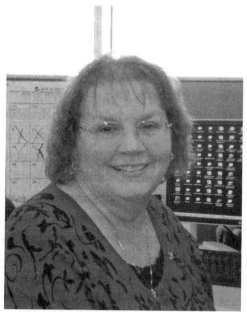

Peggy Baker, Senior Business Analyst, Reebok International.

One constant during Peggy's time at Reebok has been the beautiful office buildings, replete with all sorts of amenities, including a high-end corporate gym with all the bells and whistles, offered up to employees and their spouses at a cut rate. While this has been a perk cherished by many, for Peggy, it was like having a permanent discount at a clothing store where all the sizes are too small. She and the gym didn't quite fit:

I have tried every January, like the rest of the world, to put on my shoes and go to the gym, and it just has never stuck. I don't know if I even make it through January. I know I don't. We are so lucky ... the gym is open from six in the morning to seven at night. Literally no excuse. ... But I just always found it very solitary. I've always been overweight, and I never wanted to put on clothes to wear to the gym. I didn't want people to see me. And I always felt like I was going to be judged. That was my own opinion. So I would walk on the treadmill, I'd put my headphones on, I'd watch the TV that was attached to the treadmill, and somebody beside me would be running and I was thinking 'I hope that guy doesn't sweat on me, cause I don't really like sweat.'

When Reebok partnered with CrossFit and created a second top-notch facility for these new workouts, Peggy was not interested. Even after the buzz had permeated the walls in Canton, Peggy ignored the frenzy, feeling that the CrossFit craze was "not for me." Even when Reebok President Uli Becker encouraged her to try CrossFit, Peggy resisted. One day in the cafeteria, he pulled her aside and told her she absolutely needed to try it. He told her that it would affect her brain, make her think better, make her feel better—that it would simply make her better all around. He told her there weren't just physical benefits but emotional and mental as well. Peggy argued that she was different from the people who were able to do CrossFit, that she wasn't physically able to do something so rigorous. Uli did not relent and, after some playful negotiating as to how much life insurance money her husband would receive if she were to die trying, Peggy ultimately agreed to attend a CrossFit class. She told her husband that she was doing it to "get Uli off my back" but had no intentions of continuing. Her husband actually tried two classes with her but decided it wasn't for him. He tells her now that when he stopped he was sure Peggy was going to stop with him. It didn't happen that way.

"On-ramp" is a term used in many CrossFit gyms for the series of classes for beginners to learn the basic movements in a safe and structured way. Since on-ramp programs are made up of people new to the program, new CrossFitters can go through the series together, learning side by side in a supportive environment. Peggy vividly remembers her first day of on-ramp, when the workout included a run outside of the gym:

The coaches and people that I had known, whether for one day or twenty years, were all so different in the box. It was, "You can do it, let's do it." There was no "That's the president of the company," and "That's the security guard," and "You just work in IT." It was literally different from the very first minute. Immediately. When I came back from running ... and I came up to the box, everybody, everybody was out there cheering me on. ... I was embarrassed and overwhelmed. And when I looked at their faces—that was real. It was such a real feeling. And I thought, "Oh my God, this really is different."

Experiences that are different often make us fearful, taking us out of our comfort zones and shaking up our internal landscapes. Even when our conscious mind categorizes the experience as positive, our unconscious mind can signal danger, as the new opportunity threatens the status quo of our worldview. For fifty-three years, the forces within Peggy had labeled her as overweight, and she had convinced herself that she was unable to attain a healthy level of fitness. She could have easily told herself that the welcoming experience she'd had at her first on-ramp class was a fluke and that if she were to continue, she would inevitably feel the kind of humiliation and failure she had experienced in the past.

Bravely, Peggy went back to on-ramp classes over and over again, continuing to have that same welcoming experience she had on day one. By the end of the on-ramp series, she felt genuinely close to her cohorts and now states that the connection was "literally the strongest bond I have felt since I've worked here." Fueled by the power of this connection and comforted in knowing she would be supported and not ridiculed, Peggy chose a regular CrossFit class and ventured out of the on-ramp womb. She has never looked back. Fifty pounds lighter, with a new wardrobe, Peggy is invigorated. Her daily insulin dose has gone from eighty units to twelve, and she is on path to being free from insulin injections altogether. But the workouts alone have not led to these dramatic changes. Peggy has taken seriously the nutrition education at the Reebok CrossFit gym and has adopted the Paleo diet. She no longer struggles to eat this way—the results are motivation enough.

Like the others at Reebok with whom I spoke, Peggy is sure that the effect of doing CrossFit with coworkers has allowed for the best kind of bonding the company has ever experienced. Peggy notes that her IT team of six, who have known each other for at least ten years, is now a "tight-knit" group for the first time. "We never had this kind of relationship." In the cafeteria, people who have said a passing "Hi" for years are now asking to sit with each other and engaging in real conversation. Admittedly, the conversation often starts with CrossFit, but "it doesn't have to stay there. ... I've had real, true conversations with people who have only been a "Hi" in the past." These emerging relationships have influenced the overall work environment at Reebok, and Peggy believes it's a better place for having a renewed sense of connection and community among employees and senior management.

Peggy's own work performance has been impacted in surprising ways. In the past, when coworkers needed a Blackberry fixed, Peggy would have them deliver it to her desk. Now she finds out where they work and walks to their desk. This is a huge leap for someone who spent much of her working life sitting in a chair avoiding the few flights of stairs to the offices above. Peggy is more focused and able to work more efficiently: "I think that there's some kind of chemical thing happening in my head."

While any exercise program might have produced the benefits that Peggy has experienced through CrossFit, there is something about CrossFit's support system that made Peggy finally stick with the program and has inspired her beyond those moments of self-doubt. Walking on a treadmill is not only less transformative physiologically than the CrossFit regimen but is also emotionally unsustainable if you are wondering all the while what people think of you as the fat person on the machine.

Peggy has her own thoughts about CrossFit at Reebok and how it differs from anything she had ever tried before:

It's the coaches and how they speak to you and instantly make you feel. [The coach] stood in front of us and before we ever started ... he told us we'll be a community by the time we're through. ... We are all working for the same thing. ... That was almost the only thing he said and then the next thing you know you're running and the people are there cheering you on. Instantly, everybody in the room was watching and helping everybody else. ... People were with people they had seen for years and never even knew. You were in this separate little world. ... They say it's a cult now here ... and that's OK. I don't have any problem with that, as long as anyone can come in. It's fine with me. There is not one person that couldn't be included in it. I think it started with the very first conversation ... and instruction and going around the room and making sure every single person knew what they were doing. And never, ever once did I feel like I couldn't raise my hand. I never felt stupid or uncomfortable. Never, ever since the second I walked in that door—other than that very first run when I was afraid I wasn't going to make it back alive—have I felt insecure.

In fact, Peggy now feels more secure in her surroundings and in her own body than ever before. Part of this security is due to the new community that has sprouted up at work. She became even more aware and appreciative of this new connectedness when she attended the CrossFit Games in July of 2011 as a guest of Reebok. During the months leading up to the Games, Reebok announced that it would send two employees to Carson with the rest of the Reebok contingent. Those two employees would be chosen by lottery from a pool of people who exercised four times a week for at least thirty minutes at a time. Peggy made sure that she would be eligible for the prize, and even though her name was not one of the two drawn, the higher-ups from the CrossFit department at Reebok recognized Peggy for her great efforts and rewarded her with a trip to the Games. She enjoyed every minute of it, deeply moved by a feeling of connection to something even greater than the CrossFit community at Reebok. Peggy felt a powerful connection with others from around the country and the world who shared this culture of self-improvement.

Over the years as an owner of four CrossFit affiliates, I have spoken with many individuals about what CrossFit has done for them and most agree that their only regret is that they didn't find CrossFit sooner. Having started CrossFit myself at age thirty-eight, I echo those sentiments. So when I spoke with Peggy Baker, I was not surprised when she said, "My one regret is ..." What came out next, however, was different from what I had expected and, frankly, far more profound and touching:

> *My one thought when I'm quiet or I'm in my car or I think about this experience—I always wish my parents were alive. That's my big thing. I wish my parents could see me. I'm sure that they had wished this for me. ... I know they did.*

What more is there to say? When I asked Peggy if there was anything we hadn't covered, she added: "Did I tell you how lucky I am? I know I'm lucky. I'm lucky to work at a company that supports this so well."

The BOKS Program:
Reebok, Moms, and the School Community

In 2008, Kathleen Tullie was a full-time working mom who had been part of the corporate real estate world for eighteen years. Kathleen had two kids, ages five and eight. She lived the busy life familiar to many moms who juggle the demands of a full-time day job in heels and business suits with the challenges of being a mother. Already questioning whether this was a sustainable path for her as her kids grew and their childhoods careened by, Kathleen got a wake-up call that would urge her to make a life change. She was diagnosed with melanoma and for weeks after receiving the news, she was "paralyzed" by her fears and worries about her children, their well-being, and their future. This wake-up call combined with a combination of other life circumstances for Kathleen: "I was like 'OK, what the heck am I doing being corporate mom and working so hard and missing out on my kids?' I want to be a stay-at-home mom or do something that is going to have a positive effect on this world. And more so for my kids." This frightening event was a catalyst to try something she had been contemplating for years: to start her own business while being a stay-at-home mom.

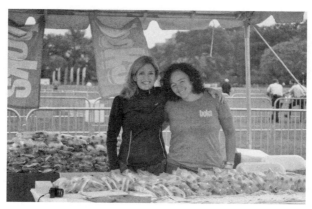

Kathleen Tullie (left) and Cheri Levitz (right)—two of the founders of BOKS at the Nickelodeon Worldwide Day of Play on the White House lawn. October, 2011.

After Kathleen's health stabilized, she was eager to contribute in some meaningful way. Always fascinated by books related to psychology, in early 2009 Kathleen stumbled upon *Spark*, written by John Ratey, M.D.[41] The book outlines the physiological relationship between brain functioning and exercise. The message to readers is compelling: physical activity leads to sharper and clearer thinking, stronger memory, and other cognitive benefits. Dr. Ratey specifically highlights the educational impact that morning physical activity can have on children. It was this part of Ratey's work that resonated most with Kathleen:

I thought, You know what? Every morning in front of my house, I have all the neighborhood kids playing soccer before the school bus. Why don't I and some other moms just go to the school and everybody can drop off their kids, and we'll be the babysitter and watch the kids play, because kids deserve to play and start their day off with a healthy start. And here's this book that's saying that kids will perform better academically, depression is mitigated, and kids will be more confident. As Dr. Ratey states, "Twenty minutes of elevated heart rate is equivalent to taking a little Prozac and a little Ritalin."

Sometimes, an idea like this might come along, housing briefly in a mind before moving on, due to lack of time in the day or money in the bank or focus in the frontal lobe to bring it to fruition. For Kathleen, though, this idea took on a life of its own. A few months after that light bulb went off, Kathleen pitched her idea to school personnel in her local district, got their approval, and emailed the most passionate and reliable workforce she could think of: other stay-at-home moms. Within days she had a great group of committed volunteer moms who launched the program in October, less than a year after Kathleen read *Spark*. Within two days of emailing parents at her kids' elementary school, she and her crew had registered eighty kids, their targeted start-up number. The program, called FitKidz at the time, took off like wildfire.

A lot of people argued, "You know what, you're free babysitting." And I say, "Great. I don't care what we are. It's benefiting everybody." ... Within a couple of weeks, parents and teachers were sending us emails saying, "Wow you're making a huge difference in my child—they're happier, they go to bed earlier, they're excited to go to school, they're asking us to exercise on the weekends." Then I had teachers telling me that some of the nurse visits were down, kids are more confident in class, and before you knew it, through word of mouth, moms from other communities were emailing me asking how to run the program in their school. I had to laugh, because I was like "There is no program, you just show up with a little passion for exercise, kids, and a whistle around your neck! Kids love to play!"

There may have been no formal program in those early days but there certainly is now. The program is simple: Three mornings per week, one hour before school, kids get to move around and have fun. Activities are noncompetitive with the goal of keeping heart rates in a certain zone for twenty minutes at a time. The hour includes socialization, warm-up, running, relay races, or obstacle courses incorporating a skill, and cool-down with a nutrition talk. The nutrition piece was a bit of an after-thought for Kathleen but it turns out that the kids are really responding to it. Trainers teach them simple, catchy things like, "If you run your snack under water and it dissolves, it's not healthy."

Soon after starting FitKidz, Kathleen obtained 501c-3 nonprofit status, with the help of a couple of other moms who took the program as seriously as she did. It was clear to Kathleen that she and her army of suburban moms could expand the program beyond their school, and she dreamed big:

I felt like here you are in middle-class America where you have all these stay-at-home moms who all have educations, who all had careers at one point, and they're so passionate about their kids. You have all the ingredients for success. I call it Mom Equity. It's an underutilized, untapped market of moms. So I thought, "This is amazing. If we could just do this everywhere!"

Running a fitness program for an hour each morning at your kids' school is one thing. Structuring and marketing the program for expansion to other districts is another, especially when there would be no capital gains for anyone. Kathleen turned to her trusted advisors for guidance. One of the women who served on the Board of FitKidz was senior counsel at Reebok. She suggested that Kathleen inquire about Reebok's interest in sponsoring FitKidz. Reebok execs were more than happy to sponsor FitKidz, explaining that they were looking for ways to revitalize their human rights initiative and give back in a big way and that the FitKidz program would help fulfill one of Reebok's long-term goals of getting kids to exercise more. Matt O'Toole, who had met Kathleen when they were both members of CrossFit New England, explains that getting kids to move was at the forefront the company's mission as executives chartered their path:

We had brought in a lot of consultants, we had looked at a lot of options. One of the statistics that came up that just blew me away was that in the modern era of sports companies, as we have celebrated athletes and celebrated elite teams, the actual per-capita participation in exercise and sport around the world had declined. ... If you added up everything that all the big brands had spent to communicate sport, it's a daunting number ... but ... actually the result was that fewer people were moving. ... So we [decided] we have to be the brand that gets people moving and it has to be more engaging.

And, Matt believed, there's no better place to start than with young children.

Kathleen was surprised and flattered by Reebok's interest in her nonprofit, and while the offer was appealing, she hesitated for some time, unsure if she wanted the branding of a large corporation involved in this grassroots effort. Kathleen and her team researched other options, speaking to government agencies about funding, and in the end, she realized that partnering with Reebok "would give me validity and sustainability," and she also recognized that their motives were genuine and in line with her own. In September 2010, FitKidz became BOKS (Build Our Kids' Success), and Kathleen was back working in the corporate world, though this time with a philanthropic twist that made things far more palatable for her psyche.

Michelle Moorehead, head of brand strategy at Reebok, is now one of Kathleen's bosses and advocates. Her enthusiasm for BOKS and its mission is contagious:

Reebok has a long-standing commitment to the community, going back to our human rights initiative, and we were thinking about how to refresh that commitment in line with our mission and in line with the current best practice thinking about how companies can most impact their communities. Sponsoring a program like BOKS ... was the perfect answer. ... We're thrilled with the incredibly positive feedback we've received from the program—from the teachers and principals involved, to the parents and students, to our own employees who have participated as volunteers. It is absolutely changing lives, and it's incredibly rewarding to see the program deliver the desired benefits—greater physical activity, better performance in the classroom, and improved social interaction.

From its humble beginnings serving one school in Natick, Massachusetts in 2009, the program reached twenty-seven schools in 2010 and is on track to be in forty schools by the end of fall 2011. Kathleen has left behind her sweats and whistle, donning professional clothes and working at Reebok headquarters much of the time. After a year of working for no pay, her salary and those of the others running BOKS is now paid through the Reebok Foundation. The Foundation also pays an hourly wage to faculty in urban schools who serve as trainers for the BOKS program. In many of the suburban schools, volunteer moms still run the workouts. Some of the schools have garnered corporate sponsors to foot the bill for their programs, while others charge participants. In Boston, five of the schools have faculty who are donating their time to serve as trainers. The program is an anecdotal success and now a more formal study of the effects of the program is under way. Judging from Dr. Ratey's work, we are likely to see empirical data demonstrating the benefits that have been clear to Kathleen and her colleagues for some time.

Asked about taking the leap of faith to make it happen with the ability to follow through in serving our children in this important way, Kathleen credits her parents for having instilled in her a sense of confidence and belief in what is possible:

I had a mother and father who were always extremely supportive of me and constantly surrounded me with compliments, support and encouragement. I think that father-daughter connection is huge. ... When fathers make their daughters feel confident, those women end up being more successful, happier, more secure. My dad—to this day—he's always said, "Kath you can do anything you want in this world." That's the type of dad he is to me. ... Same with my mom as well. Both of my parents have always let me do my own thing, they supported me and were incredibly positive.

Kathleen's husband is equally supportive, always encouraging her to do more, to take things to the next level. He is also athletic—a CrossFitter like his wife—and is behind BOKS with a belief in the importance of fitness and athleticism for all. Kathleen's children also love her commitment to fitness for kids, though they have their moments of wishing their mom were at home more. For Kathleen, those moments resurface now and then, but the far-reaching value and impact of the time spent away from her family keeps her going.

I definitely have a lot of those moments where I'm like, this is crazy. I want to be that mom and I want that time at home. But then I think sometimes when opportunity knocks and you can make a difference and you have all the right players in place you have to do it. ... But yes, there are definitely moments, but I think that's everything in life. You always wonder.

A member of CrossFit New England, one of the largest and best-known CrossFit gyms worldwide, Kathleen is no stranger to the power of community. She calls the connection among CrossFitters at her gym "bizarre" in some ways, referring to the intensity and level of support. Much as she has seen adults transforming themselves within that community, Kathleen hopes to provide similar opportunities for the young people in our schools. She is aware that this is not an easy fix but will take time and continued effort by all involved:

It's the power of the community that's going to make this successful and that's going to make a difference in our kids. ... Studies show that obese kids don't see themselves as obese, because they're surrounded by it. Their friends are obese. Their parents are obese. We need to make a movement from the ground up here and make sure that we get back to a healthier lifestyle. ... It's not just the faculty. It's not just the schools or the teachers. It's the parents, the kids, the faculty, the government, the foundations, and the private sector, and we all have to walk the walk. ... It's going to take the whole community.

Chizzie's Story

Chizzie's father was a great guy, a likeable, kind soul with a warm circle of friends and family. He was stricken with an aggressive form of cancer in his early sixties during a time when he wanted to be out playing baseball with his grandkids. As part of his treatment regimen, doctors suggested that he hire a personal trainer, because properly monitored exercise might improve his quality of life and might even help him stay alive longer. He found his way to TJ through some friends in the community and their first session together marked the beginning of a beautiful friendship. Unfortunately, Ned lost his battle with cancer far too soon.

Shortly after her father's death, Chizzie decided it was time to get into better shape and become a healthier person. The mother of two school-aged boys, Chizzie was a part-time high school English teacher who spent much of her time after class grading papers and preparing lectures. Life was busy, she was grieving, and Chizzie had neglected her own body and fitness for some time, despite keeping up with her passion for competitive tennis. Determined to make a change, Chizzie approached TJ, asking if he could help her get going. TJ connected Chizzie with a young female trainer at the gym who combined great enthusiasm with empathy. The two worked together privately for many months, jumpstarting Chizzie's fitness program, while simultaneously making her realize how far she had to go. Chizzie was thirty-nine, on the cusp of one of those milestone birthdays that tend to motivate and inspire, if not depress. Months into her private sessions, Chizzie would watch the CrossFit-inspired group workouts TJ had started, still called The Metabolic at the time. At first intimidated by the group, Chizzie became interested, curious how she might reap the benefits of the group energy and support while still feeling comfortable enough with her vulnerabilities. Cost was another motivating factor for Chizzie, as she knew that group classes were significantly more affordable than private sessions.

Soon after Chizzie started taking classes, we became an official CrossFit affiliate. Chizzie has fond memories of the early community-building experience of circling up into large groups, using hollow poles instead of barbells to learn proper weightlifting techniques. There was comfort in being surrounded by others who were also starting something new and were similarly vulnerable but open to the possibilities of the program TJ and the other coaches were introducing. With the new movements came talk of a new way of eating, based on the Paleolithic Diet. While Chizzie was intrigued and even participated in some of the thirty-day Paleo Challenges at the gym, it wasn't until the fall of 2009, about one year after she began CrossFitting in earnest, that Chizzie decided to "jump in" and give it a real go. At that time, with TJ's help, Chizzie designed a personal CrossFit challenge, which included both nutrition and workout components. She states, "I was sick of sucking at all of the CrossFit moves, especially moves that required agility and coordination. I was just carrying too much weight." Chizzie's 100-Day Plan included a strict paleo diet, with proportions governed by the Zone system of measuring and weighing foods. Also during the 100 days, Chizzie adhered to a CrossFit workout cycle of three days on, one day off.

Chizzie's experiment quickly yielded results. After about a month, she felt better, her energy levels increased and were more consistent throughout the day, she was sleeping better, she stopped getting eye infections she tended to have regularly, and her dentist noticed a marked decrease in plaque buildup. After two months, people consistently commented on her weight loss and the fact that her clothes were getting looser. Sometime in the first couple of months, Chizzie noticed a huge change in her fitness level during a tennis match. She was refueling throughout the match with oranges and nuts and never lost any energy. Despite the changes in her diet, "At no point did I feel deprived in terms of food. I found myself being more creative and thoughtful in my food choices, and more aware of what my body needed. When I knew I needed sustained energy over a long period of time, I ate protein; when my mind started fading, I ate fat; when I became low-energy or lethargic, I ate fruits and veggies. It was refreshing to feel like my body was a machine that worked effectively when properly fueled."

Despite the obvious progress Chizzie was making, it took her approximately sixty days before she felt confident enough to start taking risks at the gym. This included using heavier weights when weightlifting and higher boxes for box jumping, as well as tackling the full extension of movements that she'd previously modified. She became more and more comfortable in relying on the support of her classmates, feeling a deepening connection to the regulars at the 5:15 AM classes she attended. Although not necessarily social with these people outside of the gym, they were fast becoming good friends, confidantes, and cheerleaders, and Chizzie counted on them for encouragement and support. These relationships continued long after her 100-day challenge ended and are thriving over a year later, solidifying with each new workout. Chizzie feels connected to the gym community and feels she is part of a team at TJ's Gym, even though she does not compete at CrossFit.

Another important aspect of Chizzie's success and connection to the gym is her participation on the online discussion board. Although she has not met some of the people behind the posts, she diligently reads the daily check-ins and believes that they have enhanced her commitment to the community, allowing her to follow the progress, success, and struggles of the other CrossFitters at TJ's. She has both supported others and been supported by them during times of challenge, and for that she is clearly grateful.

Chizzie noticed other, less expected, changes during her 100-Day Challenge. Her creativity, thinking, and problem-solving skills all seemed enhanced. Her moods were more regulated and she tended to be calmer, more in control, and more easygoing than she had been before. The biggest benefit for Chizzie, however, has been the increase in self-confidence. She feels good about how she looks and what she has accomplished: "This practice in self-discipline showed me that I am still capable of pursuing and achieving personal and athletic goals beyond the age of forty. I feel like I represent a very large constituency of women in our community who give up on their body and fitness at a certain point, using 'too busy with kids, family, work, etc.' as their reason for not caring or changing. While sacrifices have been made to achieve the results I did, I hope more importantly showing others that you can change your health and fitness will be motivational."

During her 100-Day Challenge, Chizzie lost 35 pounds, (180 to 145), increased the height of her box jump max by 10 inches (12 to 22), was able to hold a handstand against a wall for the first time, and took seven minutes off of her two-mile run time (23:43 to 16:50).

Brian's Story

Brian was thirty, married, the father of a two-year-old boy, living in Marin and working in website construction. He spent most of his days sitting at his computer. In July 2008 a friend from high school who was a Navy SEAL had started doing CrossFit and Brian thought the program sounded "fun." Driving home one day, stopped at an intersection, he looked up and saw the TJ's Gym/CrossFit sign. He felt he had no excuse not to try it, considering how close the gym was to home and how often he'd be driving by.

When Brian had his introductory session with TJ, he listened intently about the program and was intrigued. He figured he would come to the gym once a week to supplement what would be an at-home CrossFit regimen in a garage gym. He had spent the Fourth of July weekend with his family in Lake Tahoe and had one of those wake-up calls that people often have but also often ignore. During a two-minute swim at altitude, Brian thought he was going to die. "I'm going to fix this permanently," he remembers thinking. At the time his fitness pursuits included the occasional golf game and backpacking trip, but there was nothing consistent or challenging going on. Overweight and out of shape, Brian had been given the following assessment at a routine physical a few months before coming to the gym: "You're in great shape. You could stand to lose a few pounds, but overall your health is fine." By July, Brian knew that this was not the case and that he had to make changes. In fact, he had quite a bit of weight to lose, and his activity level was well below what it should have been.

After his first few CrossFit classes at the gym, Brian realized that his plan to work out independently at home would mean forgoing all that the group experience had to offer. Working out with others, with

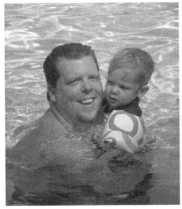
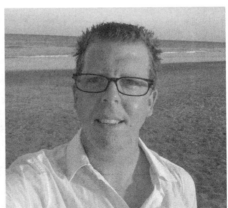

Brian Doll pre-TJ's Gym, 2007.   *Brian Doll in 2011.*

a running clock and the energy involved made it all click for Brian. He became a TJ's Gym regular, averaging four to five times each week. He was hooked, realizing he wanted to be "doing this forever," and that there "was no going back." The hardest part initially was struggling with how out of shape he was. "I could barely finish the workouts, even though heavily modified. Every class was a challenge. The physical work was hard. It was easy to want to do it, and it was easy to get to class. It wasn't easy to walk up or down stairs." Brian was so engaged by his newfound CrossFitting that he was online constantly, searching the CrossFit main site and all things CrossFit. In his online travels, he quickly learned about the importance of nutrition and knew it was only a matter of time before he jumped into that aspect of the program. Still, he figured he wasn't eating all that unhealthily, having meals like whole-grain pasta with turkey sauce. In August of 2008, just weeks after stepping foot into TJ's Gym for the first time, Brian starting following the paleo diet. Results were immediate. In the first six months, he lost fifty-two pounds. A few months later, he was down another twenty, for a total of seventy pounds. He looked like a different person and felt like one too. After his first year at TJ's, Brian documented the following results:

Lost 70 pounds of fat
Dropped cholesterol level by 26 points (13 percent)
Dropped triglyceride level by 72 percent (170 to 47)
Nearly doubled HDL ("good cholesterol") from 38 to 57
Waist size went from 38 to 31

Over time Brian has maintained his commitment to his health and fitness, and three years after starting at TJ's Gym, he is still a regular in classes and a follower of the paleo diet. He reports that his experience as part of a CrossFit community has affected his job performance, his family relationships, and his problem-solving skills.

Perspective, patience, and priorities. A favorite thought of mine is after a workout, thinking ... "This is the toughest thing I'll do all day. No matter what comes up later, I know it will be easier to manage than that workout was." I'm more patient with my team and probably with my friends and family. I feel more "centered" I guess, so I don't feel as pressured to assert an opinion as I used to. Having a consistent focus on my physical fitness means that it plays a role in how I prioritize the way I spend my time. I need to be active, so that is a big priority. I want to enjoy my time with my family, and I try to think of ways for us to be active together.

As for the lasting, global transformation of Brian, his own words eloquently describe how his world has expanded while his waistline has shrunk:

We are humans that exist in physical form. It's funny to say it that way, but at the end of the day, we exist as physical beings. I've been writing software and working with computers for almost twenty years now. The joke is that programmers see their body as a thing to move their brain around from place to place. I had a very active intellectual life as well as a very active social life, but I had no active physical life, at least not a purposefully physical life. Everything a human does involves some sort of movement, some sort of physical activity. During my intro, TJ used the phrase "physical machine," indicating that it was somewhere behind my gut. ... Being aware of my own human machine, and training it to be a well-performing human machine, literally affects everything I do. I breathe easier. Everything seems achievable. The possible just got a whole lot bigger.

Chapter 10

The Recovery Community:
Easier with Others Than Solo
Better with Exercise Than Without

Studies show that exercise has positive benefits for people with addictive disorders now in recovery. Regular exercise appears to mitigate many risk factors commonly contributing to addictive tendencies, including depression, anxiety, and stress. Exercise also has direct effects on brain chemistry, providing endorphin highs that are similar to those sought out by addicts when they reach for substances. Further, exercise can help relieve some of the symptoms of withdrawal during the detox phase of treatment. Most experts agree that some form of exercise should be included in the treatment of addictions, as a way of increasing the chances of long-term recovery, as well as boosting one's overall health, wellness, and psychological well-being.

We all know that one's ability to stick with an exercise program is variable, perhaps just about as variable as one's ability to commit to a recovery plan to overcome an addiction. I can add anecdotal evidence from my experience with many CrossFit newcomers who have quit other exercise programs but stayed with CrossFit. As we have seen, the community component of CrossFit is one of the factors that increases the probability of long-term success for its participants, enhancing both the physical results and the overall psychological experience. Similarly, addiction recovery is more likely to be successful when people are engaged in a treatment program involving the support of others outside of their treatment team.

The Twelve-Step model, most commonly seen in Alcoholics Anonymous (AA), is a well-known example of how community support facilitates recovery and how camaraderie and relational accountability can help keep recovering addicts free from substance abuse. Inpatient rehab programs almost always include a group therapy component because of the benefits of this interaction and support. For many individuals struggling with addiction, their drug of choice has been replaced by human relationships as a source of connection and feedback. A goal of recovery is to build healthy, interpersonal relationships so that the substance loses its attraction and hold, replaced by human interaction.

You can probably guess where this leads: If exercise helps recovery and group support helps recovery, how about creating a program that excels at both exercise and community. How about making use of CrossFit as one component in the treatment of addictive diseases. I'm not the first to have thought of this. The *CrossFit Journal* has included stories of former addicts who credit CrossFit with saving their lives and giving them a focus, a sense of purpose, and a support system to help them become—and stay—clean. My research on the subject led me to a website for an intriguing program called Integrative Recovery.

On a Mission: Ron Gellis, PhD

Ron Gellis is sixty-three years old. He qualified to compete at the CrossFit Games in 2011 in the sixty-to-sixty-five age division. Ron found CrossFit in 2008 through his son, who is in the U.S. Navy and who uses CrosssFit to help him stay fit. Former Navy himself, Ron has always been athletic and he took to CrossFit immediately. Despite being much older than the clientele at the gym where he began, Ron stuck with it and has experienced many fitness and emotional benefits since those first workouts three years ago.

Ron has been a licensed psychologist for more than thirty years. During most of his career, he has specialized in the treatment of addictive disorders, a path fueled by his own struggle with alcoholism and eventual recovery. Ron has directed and worked at many treatment programs around the country during his time in the field, and he has years of experience helping people reclaim their lives from the grasp of substance abuse. Ron has been convinced for some time that any effective addiction treatment program must include an exercise component. He set up a running program for prisoners with substance abuse problems, and he included scuba diving and calisthenics for adolescents battling addictions. Ron even credits exercise for helping in his own recovery and its sustainability.

Still, Ron knows that exercise alone does not provide for a comprehensive approach to recovery. He cautions against a kind of obsessive use of exercise as an attempt to overcome addiction and knows firsthand the failures of this approach. At one point when he was much younger and still struggling with his own addiction, Ron became an obsessive runner, running twenty marathons and pounding the pavement daily in order to avoid drinking. While the substitution of one addiction for another may last for some period of time, the underlying problem does not disappear and should be addressed. "You can't outrun, outpace, or outdistance the addictive disease." Ron points to the examples of professional athletes whose training and focus on exercise do not prevent substance abuse problems. "Exercise, in and of itself, for most, is not going to provide the kind of qualitative recovery that an integrated approach will offer you." For Ron, that integrated recovery came when he was forty-two years old and started attending AA meetings. With the help of his sponsor, he worked the twelve steps and found a community of support. He also figured out how to incorporate exercise in his recovery program in a more balanced way, without avoiding the underlying issues.

Just as Ron cautions against the substitution of obsessive exercise for substance abuse, he also warns recovering addicts that they might have a negative experience at many gyms: "There are a lot of rehabs that will include some sort of exercise. They'll affiliate at some Globo gym. … The typical pattern is they'll walk in. They … probably won't connect with anyone, and they may or may not do any of the exercising, and at the very best what they've done is they've had a relationship with a machine. It wasn't a personal connection."

This kind of impersonal workout is far less likely to be sustainable or transformative. Instead, Ron recommends CrossFit for his clients in recovery. As director of a thriving addiction treatment program in Southern California called Pacific Hills, Ron has incorporated CrossFit into the treatment plan for clients in both the inpatient and outpatient rehab divisions. Ron has partnered with two affiliates near his facility, CrossFit Redemption and CrossFit Orange County, where there are classes specifically for clients in recovery. Ron also directs the company's other location, Covenant Hills, in Texas, where clients attend Comal CrossFit for their workouts. Ron's program requires attendance at CrossFit classes but not participation. He realizes that each individual must make a conscious choice to accept what is offered, but he does require them to show up and observe what is going on. Their exposure to the physical workouts and the clear relational benefits of the workout community often serve as a catalyst for participation, even when clients are reluctant to join in at first. In conjunction with their sixty-day (or more) inpatient stay, which

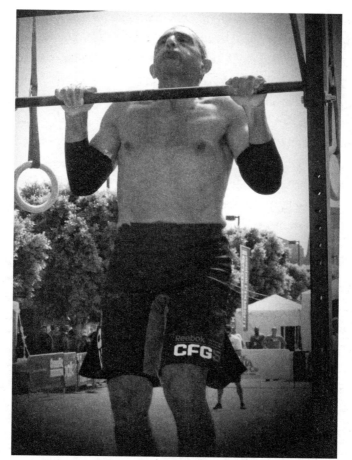

Dr. Ron Gellis competing in the Master's competition at the CrossFit Games, July, 2011, Carson, CA.

includes working the twelve steps, Ron's clients become part of not one but two communities of support.

Prior to his work as director at Pacific Hills, Ron had started a website called "Integrated Recovery," which is how I found him. Here is an excerpt from Ron's "About" page:

> *Integrated Recovery has combined the traditional aspects of 12 Step Recovery with the CrossFit methodology of fitness and nutrition (see crossfit.com). Recovery is a four dimensional*

experience encompassing the physical, mental, emotional and spiritual qualities of a person. When you start to implement the techniques and ideas taught in this program your whole life will change. It won't be overnight, but it will change. It is not magic, just practical thought processes and philosophies put into ACTION: "A Day at a Time." We strive to bring ELITE RECOVERY to the masses, one person at a time.

In an effort to provide support to more people than he could otherwise reach, Ron, feeling like somewhat of a dinosaur, has braved the terrain of social media and Internet technology. He was particularly motivated to help serious athletes and first responders (law enforcement, emergency services, firefighters), whose jobs or pursuits required a certain level of physical fitness and whose addictions, when present, might prevent them from optimal functioning. Ron offered daily blog posts that served as online meetings for those who might need such check-ins but didn't have access to meetings in person, especially military personnel on active duty. Integrated Recovery also served as a resource for those seeking treatment options. People would contact Ron, and he would refer them to appropriate treatment programs and a CrossFit gym in their area.

Since Ron became the director at Pacific Hills, he has incorporated his idea of an integrated approach into the treatment protocol at the center. He continues to field calls and emails from individuals worldwide who seek help in their battle with substance abuse. Typically, people find Ron because of their familiarity with CrossFit and their knowledge of it as a community force. Events like the CrossFit Games, according to Ron, demonstrate what CrossFit might offer them: "The power of the Games and CrossFit ... that's the ultimate manifestation of a community at large coming together. ... I get calls from people all over the world who are familiar with CrossFit and also have an issue with addiction. We are a very powerful, dynamic community which offers the support to come out of one's state of isolation and be restored to a state of health and happiness." Ron has a renewed passion for publicizing the CrossFit/twelve-step treatment model as an effective approach to recovery. He is now spreading the word on Facebook and hopes to reach even more people in need of a sustainable recovery option. Ron does not charge for his services at Integrated Recovery and considers this aspect of his work as a pro-bono "triage entity," helping people find the help they need.

Ron is driven to help others break the cycle of addiction that plagued him for much of his young adult life. Given his personal background and his professional experience, he is in a good position to accomplish this. He knows that recovery means promoting change in four dimensions—physical, mental, emotional, and spiritual, and he has experienced how each of these dimensions can be helped by CrossFit. In describing the benefits of CrossFit as part of an integrated treatment approach, Ron explains:

> *Addictive people are obsessive people by nature. CrossFit is a good, healthy hobby to participate in. It's not the only one, but it's the one that offers a wonderful community. ... For restoring one's body and mind to a state of health, CrossFit is a great exercise model and the community makes it that much more icing on the cake. My belief is, if addiction is at some level the epitome of a state of isolation ... which it is, then being a part of a healthy community is the antithesis of the state of isolation. One of the things that has made AA so successful is its sense of community, the support they can get from it. Similarly, CrossFit ... is a community, and that's a great thing.*

Jeff Hughes and Nick Cordovano: Partners in Exercise and Recovery at CrossFit Orange County

Jeff Hughes owns CrossFit Orange County (CFOC) with his wife, Robin. Like many CrossFit affiliate owners, Jeff has a second job, in his case as a firefighter. He recognizes the importance of fitness in his role at the firehouse as much as in his role as a CrossFit coach.

Jeff was acquainted with Ron Gellis and his work in addiction recovery prior to Ron's appointment as director of the program at Pacific Hills. Ron had approached Jeff early in 2011 about the possibility of CFOC playing a role in his Integrated Recovery mission. For Jeff, the answer was an easy yes: "I had already bought into the idea behind integrated recovery, meaning that I truly believe that diet and exercise can assist folks who are trying to get over that insult on their body for however many years prior." In fact, Jeff had tried to connect with an AA program in the same business complex as his gym, encouraging the clientele to utilize his services as part of their recovery process. Unfortunately, the response was poor and he was seen as just another guy trying to drum up business.

Jeff's desire to help those in recovery was based on a conviction that exercise can make a difference. So when Ron asked him to be part of the Integrated Recovery program at Pacific Hills, Jeff was eager to sign on despite the low pay involved: "The pay is inconsequential— I'm not making a killing on this by any means. ... The motivation is getting the folks that are going through their recovery to come in to get the exercise."

In the eight months since CFOC has offered classes to clients in recovery, Jeff has become increasingly convinced of the benefits of exercise for this population. Beyond the physical and physiological effects, including changes in brain chemistry, Jeff is keenly aware of the positive impact of pushing through a difficult workout. When

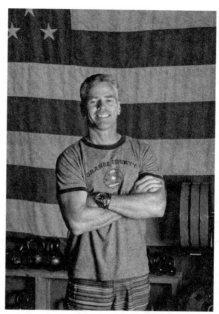

Jeff Hughes, Owner of Orange County CrossFit.

a client wants to give up during a rigorous workout, Jeff turns these moments into teaching ones:

My main message to the people is ... when the going gets tough you stick it out. ... I'm not a psychologist. I'm not anything but a firefighter and a trainer. ... When people just choose to give up because things get difficult, I think there is a real benefit from sticking it out. So if you have a physical limitation and you need to reduce the weight, or you need to reduce the amount of reps because maybe you haven't exercised in twenty-five years and you're deconditioned—fine. We're going to go really light, we're going to do half the reps. You're going to finish it in just a couple of minutes. But by God, this is the plan and it's going to be difficult, and you're going to get to the finish line and that's really the key. That to me is as important a message as doing the hard work: When the work gets tough you don't just quit.

Jeff instills this attitude of perseverance and grit in his athletes with each workout, regardless of their ability level or initial motivation. He is committed to all of his CrossFit athletes, but the element of determination has greater meaning for the clients in recovery. They typically have much to learn about the power of sticking with a program and working toward a goal day in and day out. The workouts are a good barometer of their commitment and allow them to feel the success and exhilaration that can come with even the smallest of victories, like completing a run or doing one more rep of a barbell movement.

This aspect of CrossFit training has been particularly powerful for Nick Cordovano, a graduate of the Pacific Hills program who had just completed ten months of sobriety when I spoke with him about his workouts at CFOC. Nick spent a month in rehab, attending classes three times a week with Jeff and other inpatients. Nick admits that he resisted CrossFit at first because it was "just too hard." His body went through many difficult changes during the initial recovery phase. Nick's tune changed quickly, however, as he experienced almost immediate positive results:

Me being an alcoholic, I'm all about results and being impatient with a lot of things. If I don't see results of something, I give up. I want to see something right away, and when that doesn't happen I ... give up on it. ... It didn't take long to see results doing this program—a muscle showing here or a muscle showing there. That was enough for me to be like "Wow, this is good. I feel good." That's a huge part of it, the endorphins that go on. It really boosts your confidence, and being in recovery at first we don't have much. And my self-esteem, because it's like if I do this I can start looking good again, so that built up.

And our self-esteem is in the pits when we come in. So right there are two huge things for me.

With each workout, Nick proved to himself that he could face an obstacle and persist. Upon completion of his time in rehab, Nick continued working out at a local gym, implementing aspects of CrossFit into his routine and becoming more muscular than he had imagined he could in his forties. Ultimately, Nick found his way back to Jeff and CrossFit Orange County, remembering a promise Jeff had made to him when he completed the Integrated Recovery program. Jeff had told Nick, as he tells all of the athletes in recovery when they move on from Pacific Hills or the Integrated Recovery program, that they are always welcome at CFOC, as long as they continue to do what it takes to sustain recovery:

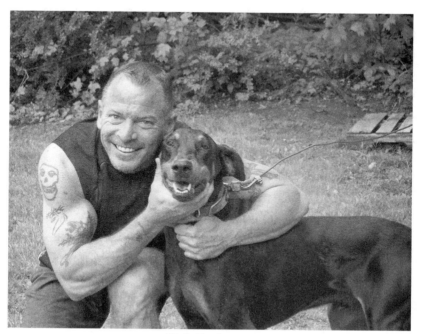

Nick Cordovano

I extend [the offer] that if you are clean and sober and you have finished with the program and want to continue to stay healthy, there is always a spot in my gym for [you]. ... I believe in the program, and I want to help these folks. ... I've met these people and I've had a very small part in their recovery, and if I can continue to help with that and say they couldn't afford it—why put a price tag on it, when the more important thing to me is for them to be healthy and recovered? ... The money doesn't matter. If I can help you, and you want to continue on, you keep coming back and I'll take care of you.

So far, Nick is the only person who has taken Jeff up on his offer. Far too many graduates have relapsed, a fact that both saddens and frustrates Jeff. He commends people who work in the recovery field for their perseverance in the face of such disappointment. He has a hard time when he has connected with a client and later finds out that he has relapsed, especially when the individual seemed to be doing well and making progress in the sobriety battle. The good news is that Nick's commitment to recovery continues, in part because of the benefits of pushing through a tough workout:

Jeff will push you to your limit. ... When you think you're going to quit, you just keep going, and the amount of confidence that gives you is unbelievable. Because in recovery, it's very easy for us to get down on ourselves. By doing this—exercising—it just gives you an incredible sense of well-being, which is really huge. ... I see now the benefit [of exercise] in recovery, in staying sober, and having it be part of my everyday program— going to a meeting, calling my sponsor, but also CrossFit. ... I feel awesome. I look good, I feel good. It gives me a sense that I can do this. I can stay sober. I can get in shape. ... I was recently laid off from work ... and I could be so down about it,

*... but I got right back into this here, and everything is good. ...
It's really because of here and doing what I'm doing that I'm
able to deal with things on a more healthy level.*

Nick is grateful for the role that Jeff, Robin, and the other athletes
at CFOC have played in his fight for recovery. He gives back by
donating time to clean the gym and doing whatever chores are needed.
He feels this is small payback relative to all that he has gained by
being part of the CFOC community as he reclaims his life from the
grasp of alcoholism:

*The support is amazing. ... It's not only Jeff and Robin ... but
the other people doing CrossFit, as well. People who aren't in
recovery. I'm here with them going through this whole thing. It
gives you such a sense of community and accomplishment. We
may not do it at the same level and get done at the same time,
but it gives us a sense of belonging. Also, being an alcoholic—
growing up was a sense of not belonging, of not fitting in. This
really gives none of that, which helps tremendously. Because
we're all doing the same thing, and we're all pushing ourselves
to the limit, and that just gives you a bonding kind of thing
[sometimes] without even knowing the other person.*

That "bonding kind of thing" is what keeps coming up in these
stories—the often unspoken connection that arises from a shared
drive and hard work. It manages to bring people together across
socioeconomic, age, gender, and other lines. How inspiring it is to
hear how Nick, with the help of his community at CFOC, is taking on
alcoholism, one workout at a time.

Peter Egyed: The Comeback Kid

Like all sports, CrossFit has its fair share of rock stars—well-known competitive athletes who have demonstrated significant talent over time, especially at the CrossFit Games. Anyone who has followed the Games since the inaugural year of 2007 has heard of Peter Egyed, a competitor in all but one of the Games, barely missing out on a qualifying spot in 2011. But Peter hasn't always been on a path of fitness and accomplishment. In fact, finding CrossFit was a huge change for this former methamphetamine addict.

Peter's drug use started during his junior year of high school. He drank and smoked pot recreationally, but his habit escalated after a football injury sidelined him from the one healthy outlet he enjoyed. Peter became so disinterested in high school that he dropped out about halfway through eleventh grade. He moved out of his parents' home, got a job and went to night school. "Mixed up with the wrong people," Peter began selling marijuana and was introduced to amphetamines. After about a month of using, he began dealing, and at that point, Peter's life "went downhill quickly." He was arrested for possession of a stolen vehicle with weapons and drugs. Although released, Peter spiraled downward, leading a "self-destructive" lifestyle for another six months before getting arrested again on similar charges. This time, he was sentenced and served a year in county jail with five years probation.

During his time in jail, Peter watched the tortured withdrawal of fellow prisoners addicted to hard drugs, thankful that his drug of choice was speed with its relatively short two-week withdrawal period of nonstop sleeping and eating. Peter did some reflecting on his life while serving time, going "back and forth about whether I was going to clean up when I got out." One important modification he made in prison was starting to exercise, a change that would have a profound effect on the rest of his life.

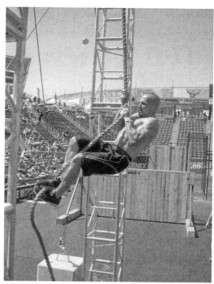

Peter Egyed, competing in the final event of the 2010 CrossFit Games, Carson, CA.

About a month after he was released, Peter found himself hanging out with the same disastrous, toxic crowd from before. He lived a drug-induced, hazy life until one fateful night when he decided to make a change. Responding to his call for help, Peter's parents took him into their home, supporting him through another drug withdrawal. During his time at home, Peter began exercising in earnest and found it to be just the therapy he needed. He wanted to quit smoking—a lingering habit—and he took up running and weightlifting. He also decided to pursue mathematics classes at a junior college nearby. Although Peter attended court-mandated group therapy sessions for drug treatment, he found this requirement tedious at best and risky at worst. Many of the people in the groups with him were not serious about their recovery, and Peter felt the meetings exposed him to potential negative influences for relapse. He found that living sixty miles from his old drug buddies was intervention enough and that exercise was the best form of treatment, so he pursued it rigorously.

After running a marathon, Peter was convinced that he was not actually fit; he didn't feel strong or physically well and was sure there must be a better way to get healthy than running long distances. When a physiology professor encouraged him to check out the CrossFit website, Peter's life changed forever. At the time, in 2006, Peter was working at the front desk of a commercial gym. He and a buddy worked out together and started incorporating CrossFit into their routine. Months later, they competed in the 2007 CrossFit Games, having had no formal coaching in the weightlifting movements. Placing 10th and so inspired by the experience at the Games, Peter knew that he had found something important in his life:

> *The Games really set in stone that this was something I wanted to pursue. Quickly, drug use or relapsing never was really in my mind. Before, I felt like it was always something you woke up and thought about—how you're going to get through the day. But soon my attention and energies were focused elsewhere. ... It was really just, "Now I have these new obstacles to overcome with these workouts" ... to this day sometimes ... people have to remind me about my past.*

Another year of training and clean living behind him, Peter competed at the 2008 CrossFit Games where the stakes were higher, the competition was harder, and the weights were heavier. He realized that his lack of access to coaching and proper equipment proved to be a disadvantage compared to the other competitors. Still, Peter managed a respectable twenty-first-place finish. Wanting to continue to improve with a goal of competing again at the Games, Peter decided to open his own CrossFit facility in Goodyear, Arizona, with a student loan and the help of his training partner. Although CrossFit Fury is now a thriving affiliate, it started simply as a way for Peter to train for the 2009 Games. He explains, "That was really the intention of opening up the gym. We would provide ourselves a place to train and hopefully build the business to support it. And now it's become a business and I have to try to find time to train." Peter's hard work paid off; his performance in 2009 earned him a sixth-place finish, catapulting him into CrossFit renown. He qualified again for the Games in 2010, finishing in tenth-place amid an extremely talented pool of athletes.

Unlike others interviewed for this book, Peter is not as quick to hail the community aspect of CrossFit. For him, it was the workouts that initially helped him stay drug-free. Later, as a CrossFit gym owner, Peter appreciated the structure and challenge of the workouts that led to something greater: "It was a pinpoint for me to focus my energies on. If it's not this, and it's not something constructive, it could be something destructive. So this gave me a direction." Much as Peter's gym started as a place for his own training and evolved into a business of training others, so did his internal focus evolve into a recognition that others depended on him and that the human relations element now mattered a great deal:

> *So now I have this community around me. ... I am a fairly solitary person. ... I try to keep things to myself, deal with things by myself. But ... I ... definitely think the fact that I'm interacting with people and helping them is a huge part of my success. ... I feel so responsible for these people ... who are relying on me to be here every day and provide a service to them, so [relapsing] is just not an option.*

While Peter's road to community was roundabout, in the end he is in a place where his connections with people are significant and meaningful. He acknowledges the impact he has on others and has accepted his role as a leader of a group sharing the goal of improved physical and mental health. Peter understands the therapeutic possibilities that lie within the prescription of CrossFit:

I do see great potential for this [CrossFit] to be a form of rehabilitation. ... It could be substance abuse, it could be PTSD, even people coming from bad lifestyles. I think having ... something to put our energy into and put our focus into that leaves us feeling gratified and satisfied and feeling that we accomplished something. I think that's what a lot of people are searching for. ... I don't even think we know the extent of how we're capable of helping people.

Dylan's Story

Growing up in rural Maine left Dylan with a lot of idle time, cruising and drinking with his buddies. On any given weekend night, they would drink until the supply was gone and then head to Denny's for some late night splendor in the form of fries and a vanilla Coke. While the crew also dabbled in pot—a highly risky activity since Maine had a zero-tolerance law for marijuana—Dylan liked drinking best, and he found it to be a good way to reward himself for performing well academically and in his after-school activities. Dylan was a good student and athlete at the small prep school he attended, so "rewarding" himself became a frequent activity.

Dylan's parents are both doctors (MD and PhD) and neither has ever struggled with addiction; in fact, there is no family history of substance abuse. Dylan continued to drink heavily in college but, "It wasn't until law school that my drinking [really] escalated. As work became harder, the celebrations got bigger. And actually, truth be told, my grades were pretty awesome." This work-reward cycle was ingrained in Dylan by the time he graduated from law school. Soon after graduation, Dylan found yet another reason to drink. His girlfriend of three years broke up with him, and he needed a way to escape the emotional pain.

It was the first time I really had my heart broken and it was the first time I ever drank to escape. I moved back to Maine, got a job at a firm, and bought a condo. I used to lie on the floor with a bottle of Jameson and listen to records and watch snowflakes melt on my skylight. I would wake up with the needle hitting the end of the record and the bottle empty. If you would have asked me then if I liked my life, I would have told you I absolutely loved it.

About a year into the life he thought he loved, Dylan decided to make a change. He moved to San Francisco to live with some friends and "start over." He got a job at a music venue in the city which was far too conducive to a party lifestyle: "Some of the best times

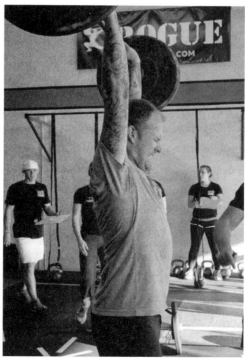

Dylan Grimes, TJ's Gym member, competing at the TJ's Games, October, 2011.

of my life were spent working at that club. I had a lot of friends and I didn't know any of their last names. We just drank, bought eight balls [cocaine], and danced with beautiful women. Not a bad way to end your twenties." But actually, it was, and somewhere deep down, Dylan knew it:

> *My friend Tom says that to be good at drinking, you have to do it every day, and that's what I did. I realized all my dreams were not wrapped up in this 365-days-a-year twenty-first-birthday-party lifestyle I had going on. And this is when the torture really started. I tried to quit and couldn't. I lost friends, girlfriends, jobs, and places to live.*

In 2007, almost three years after graduating from law school, Dylan put himself in rehab. There was no dramatic intervention—just a suggestion from a girlfriend. Dylan went on his own terms and stayed for twenty-eight days. It worked, but reentry into the world after his stay was challenging. "I had a very humbling experience after rehab. I worked in a small studio, building picture frames, and spent a good deal of time trying to get my life back on track. It was very hard." During this time, Dylan smoked often but never drank. He recalls feeling "kind of lost" during his first year of sobriety, and he was replacing alcohol with food, cigarettes, and coffee. "My sleep pattern was way out of whack and I sort of developed this depression in that first year."

Although Dylan struggled, he credits AA for providing him with a form of group therapy and the twelve steps through which he was "able to have the obsession over drinking lifted." Ultimately, another great help was physical activity. At the suggestion of a friend who had long been a proponent of exercise for people in recovery, Dylan started trail running. He hadn't run much since his college days ("It's hard to drink every day and run"), and the dormant endorphins that awoke in him felt great. Still, he didn't change much else about his lifestyle, continuing to smoke and consume more than his share of coffee and junk food.

It just so happens that the frame shop where Dylan worked during his initial recovery period was located next door to TJ's Gym. He would watch people running in and out of the building during their workouts, and he would check out what they did inside the gym from time to time, a curious onlooker with his tattoo sleeves, cigarettes, and fast-food containers. After some prodding from a friend and finding courage from within, Dylan decided to quit smoking and start taking classes.

I was instantly hooked. Exercise has been key to my sobriety. I have replaced that camaraderie I felt in bar rooms and clubs with the same feeling I get in the gym. A new WOD [workout of the day] or piece of equipment instills that same feeling I used to get when a new whiskey or beer hit my favorite local bar. ... It immediately turned my life around.

Dylan is quick to point out that the twelve steps had to come first; he could not have accepted what TJ's Gym and CrossFit had to offer had he not first worked the steps. "I needed to psychologically clean up the wreckage of my drinking years in order to progress. Now my reward is to go to CrossFit at the end of the day, which some people think is insane!" One of the aspects of the gym that had Dylan hooked early on was the ability to see progress so clearly and quickly. Like Nick Cordovano, Dylan comments on the instant gratification alcoholics crave. For Dylan, the high after a workout provides immediate feedback, while tracking his strength gains and skill development allows for long-term gratification.

Also therapeutic has been the camaraderie of the gym experience. With the support of the hundreds of people at TJ's Gym and CrossFit, Dylan has sustained his recovery and has begun the difficult process of turning his life around. He is set to take the California bar exam in 2012 and says that his recent gains in self-esteem and general feelings of empowerment come from the gym community. For the first time in years, he is "fired up about myself again." Dylan shares his thoughts about sobriety, recovery, and the forces that sustain it:

TJ's is a community of recovery. It is a community of people recovering from a society that makes it hard to take care of yourself physically after the age of thirty. A society inundated with overeating, alcoholism, sleep deprivation, abnormally high levels of stress, depression, etc. In a nutshell, we are all pretty sick, and we are all victims, until we choose to do something about it. That is the fork in the road I stood at a few years back. To the left, drown out life with a steady stream of alcohol, rock n' roll and meaningless relationships, or to the right a better life, with health, prosperity, and a certain amount of awesome unpredictability. I chose to go right [with CrossFit], and I could never have predicted how beautiful a choice that would be.

We are a community of ex-pro athletes, ex-collegiate athletes, part-time workers, full-time moms, semi-pro marathon runners, recovering alcoholics, newly divorced dads, relocated Apple employees, etc. We are so big and so deep you find one of everything in our midst. We are a group that would not normally mix. ... That is the beauty, that we get together and form this community of support that I have only seen in other recovery circles like AA. We stand and cheer for the last one moving [in a workout]. There is a saying in twelve-step programs that the most important member is the newest one. Isn't the same thing true for CrossFit? Wouldn't we die out as a community if we didn't see someone get a pull up for the first time every week? When our own goals are not enough, there is always someone else with a bigger one. I love CrossFit. It lets the rock' n roll live inside me, in a healthy way. In fact I am more rock' n roll power cleaning than I ever was doing a Jagerbomb.

Chapter 11

Team, Competition, and Community

September 25, 2001. The New York Yankees held its first home game at Yankee Stadium following the devastating attacks on our country. Psychologists, newscasters, spectators, players, and coaches alike noted the profound symbolism of that game and its impact on the psyche of New Yorkers—and all Americans. For many, there was something soothing and settling about that game; it provided a communal experience of grief and mourning while at the same time reminding us of the possibility of normalcy returning to our lives. There are numerous examples of sporting events affording a similar kind of communal solace, but that Yankee game was especially noteworthy after the enormity of 9/11.

Anyone who has ever rooted for or played on a sports team knows that there is something about team competition that brings people together. I would suggest that our penchant for identifying with a team is an outgrowth of our desire for community on a larger playing field. Few things can bring strangers together as quickly and effortlessly as flying a team's colors. Ever gone to a bar on Super Bowl Sunday? Remember the pep rallies in high school or even Sunday morning Little League games? And how about those college football games, painted faces and all? It is quite a phenomenon, really, the ways in which people come together in support of a group of athletes. The intensity and degree of affiliation are as varied as the motivations that people have for affiliating. While some choose to root for a particular team in order to feel a part of something, others might be there simply in support of a brother, sister, son, daughter, or friend, and the common ground shared with other team fans is a by-product of this individual support.

In fact, it is not just teams that can bring people together; think about Dale Earnhardt back in his day, or Chris Evert in hers. The element of sport and competition has the power to draw people together. There is something compelling and fascinating about watching athletes perform bodily feats and exert physical effort, demonstrating skill and prowess on the one hand and extreme, sustained effort on the other. We might imagine ourselves in those bodies or we might feel that the gifted athlete is an entirely different species. Almost universally, though, the experience of taking in sport in the company of others has a group-bonding effect. There are also elements of fun and shared enthusiasm, especially when your favorite team wins.

In exploring the power of community, we have heard about the common ground and bonding experiences from shared suffering or effort—whether on the battlefield, in the wilderness, through an illness or addiction, or in the gym. This mutual struggle can have the effect of bringing people together in meaningful ways. We have also seen how the intensity of CrossFit makes it likely to bring people together with similar communal connections. Part of this intensity relates to the competitive aspect of CrossFit—one of the premises of the experience is that one should track one's progress over time, thereby encouraging competition with one's self. And competition with others may be part of our DNA.

As we conclude our observations on the power of community exemplified by CrossFit, the phenomenon of CrossFit as an individual and team sport with competitions in local gyms, at regional meets and international games brings the force of connection to another level. The thing about CrossFit is that every workout performed with others is an opportunity for being a spectator/cheerleader/fan while simultaneously being a participating athlete. The CrossFit culture is infused with the expectation that you will sweat together and cheer each other on with mutual support. It doesn't matter if you're meeting for the first time or if you've been friends for years; you may expend almost as much energy encouraging each other as you will exercising. In addition to being one of those unspoken, seamlessly transmitted CrossFit traditions, this practice of competition and support may well be embedded in our psyche.

When I turned forty in 2009, I wrote an article for the *CrossFit Journal* about the nature of competing at CrossFit after a certain age. While the focus of that article was on the aging competitor, my sentiments about what drives us to compete are relevant to our discussion here:

It had been a while since my days of competing to win. While winning is nice, for most of us, the prospect of being number one in any athletic endeavor ends with the acceptance of a college diploma. When I ran marathons in my twenties, I certainly wasn't running to win. When I backpacked the John Muir Trail in the Sierra Nevada Mountain Range in my twenties, I wasn't doing it for time. When I took up snowshoeing as a winter sport, I wasn't planning on becoming a competitive snowshoer who could win races.

But CrossFit changes everything. It taps into those parts of our psyches that house competitive instincts and fuel our physical pursuits. It calls upon dormant hormones and startles to awareness the athlete in all of us. With each WOD, we are forced to decide how hard we will push, how fast we will go, how much we will lift, how well we will move. Unlike our contemporaries gliding on the elliptical machines with magazines in hand, we cannot go through the motions of our exercises while thinking about something entirely unrelated.

The intensity of CrossFitting at any level requires an internal dialogue and source of motivation that precludes distraction and disallows a half-hearted approach. It also makes us find a reason to come back and do it again the next time. Simply put, CrossFit is too hard to be a mindless endeavor. It both evokes and requires emotional commitment. Perhaps this is why it also makes us competitive, regardless of our age. After all, competition simply entails trying to do something well—better than the last time or better than someone else.

... And then there's the feeling we get when we learn something new with our bodies and try to master it in order to be better. Like drinking hot cocoa, it makes us feel young again, creating a physiological response that brings us back to our days on the soccer field with our parents cheering for us on the sidelines. Along these lines, our bodies' instinctual responses to competition—racing heart, jitters, butterflies—all hark back to the days of our youth when nerves played a major part in so many life experiences.[42]

I have felt all of these things and more when competing as part of the TJ's Gym affiliate team at the CrossFit Games in 2009, 2010, and 2011. With my parents and children in attendance at the NorCal

Regionals in 2011—the qualifying competition leading up to the Games—the emotions were heightened. It is not so much about outcomes. Of course it is more fun to win than to lose in absolute terms, or do better than worse in relative terms. Winning the 2011 NorCal Regional was definitely a high for us all, while coming in twenty-second place at the Games in 2010 was a relative low. Our eleventh place finish in 2011 falls somewhere in between. But beyond workout details, performance, and placements, the Games are simply another outlet for connection with others—teammates, spectators, and the event organizers and volunteers.

I can remember back to my competitive days on the soccer field when I felt validated and important as an athlete, aware of being a conduit for the emotions of our fans. I can remember how exciting and inspiring that was, especially when younger soccer hopefuls would express their delight in our performance and example. Appearing in the local newspaper or college weekly was thrilling and transmitted the feeling of mattering on some larger scale, however illusive and transitory. But something far more meaningful has

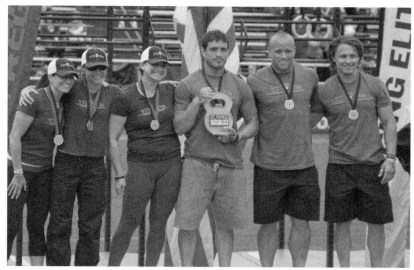

Author, far left, with her TJ's Gym teammates, NorCal Regional Champions, May, 2011, San Jose, CA.

transpired for me as a CrossFit competitor and representative of our TJ's Gym community. I know from talking with team members at other gyms that my experience is not an isolated one. Reinforced by the sponsorship of Reebok at the 2011 Games with expanded media coverage, many of us had a taste of being important to the outside world and could imagine what professional athletes experience on a regular basis. What was most tangible, alive, and important to me, however, was the experience of our team coming together in competition with the powerful support of our community; looking up into the stands at a sea of blue TJ's Gym shirts waving and cheering us on was heartwarming and motivating. If there was ever a doubt that people are inclined to rally in support of their representatives in sport, just attend a CrossFit competition at any level; the community spirit is overwhelming and inspiring.

In the spring of 2011, CrossFit held a worldwide online competition called the Open, comprised of a series of weekly workouts to be performed to given standards. Workouts could either be judged in person at a registered CrossFit gym or via video submission. Thousands of athletes competed, and each person's performance was ranked at the regional and international level. Rankings were used for qualification for Regionals—the next level of competition, both for teams and individuals.

Like many CrossFit affiliates, TJ's Gym held weekly Open workout times when athletes could come and be judged. Not surprisingly, these sessions yielded some incredibly inspiring and moving efforts. It didn't matter whether an athlete was trying to qualify for Regionals or to complete a single rep in the time allotted; no matter the goal, regardless of the level of skill and strength, each athlete was treated like a superstar. Moms of young children reclaimed parts of themselves they had not known since competing as girls on youth sport teams. Former collegiate football players pushed themselves as if they were back at that homecoming game years earlier. Adults who had been teased on the playground in grade school because of their awkwardness shed their internal "fat kid" and "kicked ass" in the workouts. All of this and more transpired amid the roar of cheers in a room filled with enough energy to power just about any human feat.

To be in the presence of that kind of emotional fuel is awe inspiring and uplifting. I heard from a number of participants about what it meant for them: the experience was nothing short of life-changing, with people relating emotional highs that were second only to the birth of a child. People spoke of family relationships becoming more intense. They talked about coming to terms with previous life failures. They spoke of breaking down perceived barriers and preparing to take on new goals in their work lives. While varied and diverse, the reflections shared a common thread: what struck people most and what made the experience so transformative was the palpable feel of support from others in the room. One of our members wrote about her experience with the Open, providing an especially powerful commentary on how her participation in CrossFit has brought her closer with her husband:

The week we did the deadlifts, Joe [my husband] was right there, talking to me and with his voice lifting that barbell with me every time. The look on his face when I was done was one I will not soon forget. CrossFit has brought us together in a way that I can't really explain. I know you know what this is because you told me this would happen, and I thank you for embracing me with open arms when I said I was ready. Joe and I have been together for seventeen years, and it wasn't until this past year that we worked out together for the first time. Crazy—especially knowing the kind of athlete he is. People have probably looked at us all these years and thought we were the most mismatched couple—but we are going strong and getting stronger together.

The Open highlighted the community aspect of CrossFit and much of what we have explored through the stories in this book. Profound and meaningful was the warmth of human support and connection through shared effort, commitment, and physical struggle. For the TJ's Gym community and hundreds of others worldwide, this high continued on through the next phase of competition at Regionals, where the playing field was larger and less intimate but no less inspiring. The final glory culminated at in the Games in Carson, California, where fifty of the world's best CrossFit teams competed at the Reebok/CrossFit Games of 2011.

I've heard from hundreds of our athletes that rallying around a team of individuals coming together and working towards an extreme physical goal was both motivating and humbling. Unlike most professional sports where the athletes are untouchable and isolated from the spectators, in CrossFit there is a much closer common experience between competitors and noncompetitors. For the most part, those who compete use the same equipment and take the same classes as those who don't. There is a common language, an appreciation for the struggle to master a movement. Shared also is the knowledge that nutrition, sleep, stress, and emotional well-being affect athletic functioning, and the challenge of integrating these elements is the same, regardless of degree of excellence. If you CrossFit with any level of commitment, you know what it's like to make sacrifices, to give up that chocolate cake or late night out with the girls. The unifying element is a greater appreciation of the sacrifice made by others, especially when those others happen to be pretty darn good at a sport you know well as both participant and spectator.

A funny thing is happening around the world of CrossFit these days. It is called a throwdown—a local competition where people from different gym communities come together and turn workouts into sport. In fact, CrossFit is expanding the idea of working out as sport, featuring personal bests and competitive challenges. If you've never been to a throwdown, you should go, if only to get a taste of the power of community displayed there. And if you go, you will see regular people doing amazing things with body and mind. If you are skeptical reading this, you may be the perfect candidate to experience the power of this collective spirit. Have you allowed yourself to be open to the friendship, support, and inspiration of others? Perhaps you just haven't found the right affinity group that might inspire you to change your life for the better, or the right activity that is both challenging and pleasurable. It might be a quieter forum than that of the CrossFit community, but the potential for connection is out there for all of us—if we are open to the power of community.

Danny's Story

At the Reebok/CrossFit NorCal Regionals in May 2011, Danny Nichols, a member of the TJ's Gym/San Rafael affiliate team, shocked spectators with his record-breaking 325-pound thruster. A thruster is a movement that begins with a barbell front squat and ends with a press overhead, all in one fluid motion. In this competition, the barbell started on the ground, so the athletes had to first do a clean (an Olympic weightlifting movement) to get the bar up and ready for the thruster. The next closest finisher worldwide reached 285 pounds. With this one lift, Danny was catapulted into global CrossFit stardom and local celebrity status, and he has since become known as the strongest man in CrossFit. With his thruster now the stuff of CrossFit legend, Danny is often approached by strangers curious about his background and training.

Danny's road to CrossFit fame has been a rocky one. Born to a teen mom who had three children prior to her twenty-first birthday (her first at age fifteen), Danny endured a difficult home life for much of his childhood. His mother left when he was two years old, in her quest to experience a life of her own as a young adult in her early twenties—at least this was the best explanation Danny has ever received. Danny

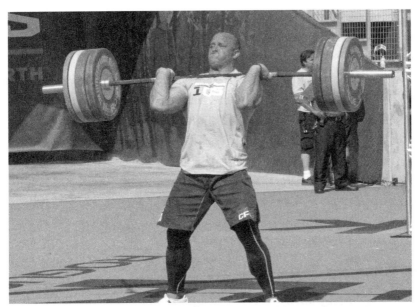

***Danny Nichols of TJ's Gym competing at the
2011 CrossFit Games, Carson, CA***

was raised by his father and two different stepmothers, along with his paternal grandmother, with relatively little contact with his mother over the years. Family life was chaotic at best and volatile at worst. Danny was a teenager when his half brother and sister were born, and he was expected to care for them much of the time. He even shared a room with his infant brother during high school—no easy task, especially with middle-of-the night feeding calls and crying spells.

As he grew, Danny found comfort in his athleticism, playing basketball, baseball, and football in middle school and high school. Team practices gave Danny a purpose, engaging him during after-school hours when he might otherwise have been getting into trouble. Academics were not his strength, as there was little structure and encouragement at home.

Graduation from high school meant reckoning with some kind of long-term goal, and Danny had his sights set on playing in the National Football League (NFL) like so many other American boys.

But Danny had a unique gift, and the dream seemed attainable. First stop was the College of Marin in the San Francisco Bay Area, where he played running back as a freshman, earning All-League honors. Upon entering his sophomore year, he was designated as Pre-season All-American, but fate would intervene three weeks prior to opening day of his sophomore season. During a scrimmage, a team member who was playing against him became angry and agitated on the field and poked his finger into Danny's helmet, puncturing his eye and severing his optic nerve. The damage was devastating and lifelong; Danny is completely blind in his right eye.

Shortly after the incident, Danny held out hope that his eye would become functional again, but after consultation with numerous specialists, he was finally forced to accept his fate. His physical and psychological recovery were painstaking, aggravated by a particularly frustrating legal process. In the end, Danny had a $50,000 settlement in return for lost vision in one eye. Depressed and angry, Danny tried to come to terms with his situation, partying often but still wanting to return to the playing field. "I knew I could either stay depressed or try to do something about it. I didn't want to be the comeback kid at College of Marin. I wanted to go somewhere where nobody knew my story, so I went down to Pasadena." Tough times continued when Danny sprained his ankle and missed the season at Pasadena Junior College, but his potential was recognized when he earned a scholarship to Minnesota State.

As close to big-time ball as Danny had ever been, his time at Minnesota State also had its ups and downs. Danny played fullback and started on every special-teams lineup, helping the team to its biggest turnaround in the history of the program. While his football success was clearly rewarding for Danny, winters in Minnesota were tough, and he missed the California climate and lifestyle. After his senior season at Minnesota, Danny left school and returned home. Danny's homecoming signaled to him that it was time to get serious about training for the NFL combine, the forum for tryouts for all NFL teams. Lacking access to well-connected agents and other networking opportunities, Danny attended the free-agent combine in 2006. Despite a great showing there, he was not picked up by any team.

Frustrated and disappointed, Danny quickly blew through the money he had received in his settlement, partying with friends, taking trips to Vegas and going on shopping sprees that served as temporary mood-enhancers. Unemployed and rather directionless, Danny moved to Los Angeles where he was introduced to bodybuilding, entering a number of competitions. His drive for athletic challenge was sorely unsatisfied, however, as was his increasing desire for a place to call home and a meaningful social circle. After two years, Danny was "burnt out on the party lifestyle and ready to start over." He yearned to live at home again, ever hopeful that life there might be different this time around. It wasn't. Danny's return to Marin in late 2009 was a difficult one: "I didn't have anything. I didn't have any money. My relationship with a girlfriend was going sour, and I just needed something." With his competitive drive still alive and kicking, and sensing that he needed a focus and structure, Danny started weightlifting and training again. He also played semi-professional football from January to March of 2010.

In the summer of 2010, a former Olympic weightlifting coach encouraged Danny to try lifting at TJ's Gym, just around the corner from his home. He started attending the TJ's Gym Barbell Club, which was right up his alley. During one Sunday session in July, Danny joined a number of athletes at the gym who were keeping a close eye on the computer, following the TJ's Gym affiliate team at the CrossFit Games in Carson. Intrigued by what he saw on the live stream, Danny tried his first CrossFit class when the team returned a few days later.

Weighing in at 260 pounds and by far the largest and strongest person who had ever completed a workout there, Danny was a spectacle even before he lifted a barbell. Once he did, he became a circus act of sorts. But Danny was no one-trick pony; it turned out that he could do far more than just move heavy weights. He could jump higher and sprint faster than anyone else. He picked up challenging skills like rope-jumping double-unders and muscle-ups (a gymnastics movement) with ease. He was clearly an incredible all-around athlete and a huge hit in classes, not only because of his feats of strength, but because of his larger-than-life personality. Danny was quickly making his presence known within the TJ's Gym community, connecting with people in exciting and new ways.

Soon after, Danny's grandmother died and he went through some personal turmoil, dropping out of the gym for some time, temporarily unable to benefit from the gym's support system. Realizing how much was there for him, he returned months later, training hard and earning his membership by helping out wherever needed. By this time, it was clear to Danny and the rest of us that he had a future in the sport of CrossFit, and he was invested in learning to become a coach and a better athlete. He shadowed TJ's classes and immersed himself in other learning opportunities, ultimately earning his CrossFit Level One Certification in June of 2011.

Danny's presence on the TJ's Gym affiliate team during the 2011 season helped catapult the team to a first-place finish at the NorCal Regionals. While the team's eleventh-place finish at the CrossFit Games in Carson was somewhat disappointing, Danny was left with a renewed sense of commitment to the training and sacrifices that might allow for a better team finish in 2012. Danny is on that path now, working to improve areas of relative weakness and dedicated to making sound nutrition and lifestyle choices that will enable him to best contribute to the team's success.

Beyond the athletic competitive outlet for Danny, what has been most transformative is the community connection he has made through CrossFit and TJ's Gym. Having experienced a tumultuous past and lack of supportive interpersonal relationships for much of his life, Danny is now an integral part of this community of athletes and coaches. Much as he is driven to succeed at the sport of CrossFit, representing his adopted family at TJ's Gym, Danny is also empowered to cultivate the relationships that have formed along the way. While finding this supportive culture and a larger affinity group wasn't his intent when he took his first CrossFit class, Danny is grateful for this welcomed by-product of his reentry into competitive sport. "At TJ's, I've found a mentor and a family and a team. I'm pretty lucky to have all of that in my life."

Chapter 12

A Perspective from Inside CrossFit Headquarters

Tony Budding

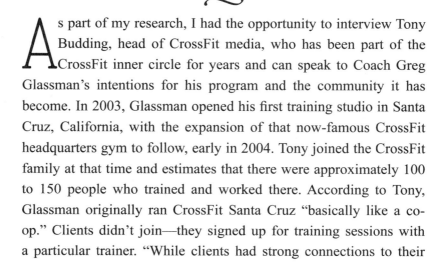

As part of my research, I had the opportunity to interview Tony Budding, head of CrossFit media, who has been part of the CrossFit inner circle for years and can speak to Coach Greg Glassman's intentions for his program and the community it has become. In 2003, Glassman opened his first training studio in Santa Cruz, California, with the expansion of that now-famous CrossFit headquarters gym to follow, early in 2004. Tony joined the CrossFit family at that time and estimates that there were approximately 100 to 150 people who trained and worked there. According to Tony, Glassman originally ran CrossFit Santa Cruz "basically like a co-op." Clients didn't join—they signed up for training sessions with a particular trainer. "While clients had strong connections to their trainers, there wasn't a cohesive feeling of 'I belong to CrossFit Santa Cruz.'"

The idea that the first CrossFit gym started as a group of not-so-connected trainer-athlete dyads is fascinating, considering how it has evolved since then. What might be most surprising to devoted CrossFitters who recognize the power of CrossFit communities worldwide, is that the community component was not created or implemented as part of any long-term business plan or design. In fact, the growth of CrossFit itself was not mapped out in any way. According to Tony, much of Glassman's decision to work as a fitness trainer in his early days had to do with the lifestyle it afforded him: "The reason he was a trainer was because he could work hard for as few hours as possible and maximize the enjoyment of his free time. He could go bike riding and hang out with his friends. He very consciously wanted the lifestyle of a trainer, but he was also really interested in the question, *What does it mean to be fit and how do you get fit—what is that?*"

Early on, though, it was clear that something was happening within the context of Glassman's workouts that would be the beginning of the community component we know today. As Budding explains:

Greg and his clients would get together regularly. He was always working out with his clients and would go on bike rides with them and have barbecues in the parking lot, so there was always that sense of "being in it together," more so obviously once they had their own gym. This is what they did naturally and it fit. There's something about the shared suffering. It's very much what he did. It wasn't a design; he wasn't thinking, "Well I'd like to have a business and probably the best way to make the business successful is to create a community." It was ... when you do these hard workouts the people that tend to like doing them and the people who tend to stick around and thrive in that environment are the kind of people you want to hang out with. So it just sort of worked out that way. It's pretty cool.

But how did the community aspect develop and why did people continue to come together and stick with the program and make these connections? Tony expands on the organic nature of the process:

This idea that like attracts like and you push hard, you keep real, and you deliver good performance that's hard. ... But look, getting in shape is really difficult. It's never been designed to be an ethical barometer but it actually is for the most part. The ethics of criminals is the easy way: impatient, short-term, immediate, least effort. CrossFit is the opposite of all of those things. ... You have to work hard, you have to tolerate discomfort, you have to put up for the long-term, and those actually are character traits of really cool people, and so why not create a community of those? But again, it's more a natural result than some kind of conscious effort. ... CrossFit makes people better. So you create this group of people about becoming better. And having fun has to be a part of it ... and having fun cements the community ...

... There's certainly an intimate connection between caring about someone else's success and building community. ... If you genuinely care, it has to happen. You have to want to be around people. We're a relationship business. If you don't like people, it's probably not a great business choice. ... We certainly value community. ... Getting fit is hard. ... If you're unfit when you start, you have to change quite a bit of your life. ... You have to commit a certain number of hours per week. ... Chances are pretty good you have to modify your diet. That's hard. Really hard. Especially if you've been eating a certain way for a long period of time, but you also have to

be willing to tolerate discomfort, you have to be willing to escalate your effort and also to moderate your effort, because it's not just going to be onward and upward. You're going to have some good days and bad days. Chances are you're going to have some kind of injury, you're going to get sick. And so it's like can you tolerate all of these things? ... You feel an automatic kinship with someone who suffers with you. We all suffer together. ... It can't be just about the workouts. So how and where does it extend beyond, outside? Where are the boundaries? When does it go from being just a gym relationship to being a personal relationship? How does that evolve? ... Someone comes in for a workout and ends up getting so much more; and what's that experience and are there common threads? ...

It's hard to pinpoint. It's human interaction. I know when I was first coming to the gym when I was a client I didn't want to leave. It was cool and there were interesting things going on. So much of this ... to get a little dramatic ... is like the human struggle. Right? Hamlet is a hero because he knows he's going to fail, but he keeps going in spite of that. We know we're going to find our limits, but we keep going in spite of that. ... There's so much BS in the world. CrossFit is so real; ... the essence of these movements has a real effect on you, and if you keep doing them you do get better and it's profound. ... That's so refreshing ... and it tends to permeate our culture too, you know, no bullshit. Community is about a shared purpose, and CrossFit is about making your life better.

Greg Glassman via the CrossFit *Journal*

Earlier, in an interview at the 2011 Games, Greg Glassman discussed the role of community in CrossFit. Video excerpts of this interview were aired recently in the *CrossFit Journal*. When asked how exercising with others and how CrossFit's social approach changes the experience and outcome for individuals, Glassman explained:

> *The major aspect that really made the difference is the camaraderie. ... Captain Michael Perry of First Special Forces Group gave me a phone call one day out of the blue, and he says, "Coach, you've taught me something critical here ... I'm an army captain, I'm an SF [Special Forces] captain and long known the importance of camaraderie, and we work for it wherever we can get it, but we've learned through CrossFit the formula for camaraderie, and I can now duplicate it anywhere. ... It's agony coupled with laughter." And I knew at once. ... "You're ... right, man, I get that." Because collapsing, sweating, complete and total physical failure, coupled with a bunch of people folded over laughing their asses off—not at the person down and out—but at something else ...*

> *It was an interaction with a group that you'd never in a million years see at [other gyms]. In that environment, you come in, you do your own workout, there might be someone you talk to at the water fountain, you may even bring your own music to tune the world out—it used to be the Walkman now it's the iPhone or the iPod ... but I knew people in the old days who would put a pair of earphones in and just stuck the other end into their pants, so no one would talk to them, just to keep people from interacting with them. ... People were there to have a singular private unique experience. They were almost like renting the space from the gym owner ... to work out by themselves. Our environment is very, very different. ... You don't have an option but to interact with others. And they will. And if they get a*

sense that you're a little bit keeping to yourself, they're going to be in your face. You're going to get bothered.[43]

When Coach Glassman says "bothered," I interpret it to mean being bothered in the sense of unsettling your status quo, of disrupting your routine in order to make a change. Bothered in the way that our psychological equilibrium is shaken up when we finally expose the long-standing behaviors we would like to change but repeat, despite our best intentions. Bothered by being prodded into the group experience, by not being left alone, by being stirred to action.

Uli Becker bothered Peggy Baker to the point where she finally joined CrossFit, and she is now fifty pounds lighter and almost insulin free. Ron Gellis bothers his clients in substance abuse treatment, making them attend CrossFit classes even when they aren't sure they want to participate. When Brad Ludden was bothered by his aunt's cancer, he started First Descents for young adults with cancer. Kathleen Tullie bothered school administrators to get them to allow her to start an exercise program for kids before school. Brad McKee bothers us all, asking that we not forget the sacrifices of our military personnel. And the list goes on.

We see that being "bothered" by others may force us out of our own head to allow change to take place. Further, if we become "bothered" enough, we may move to action and start bothering the status quo of others; the positive ripple effect is that we bother to make a difference in the lives of others, because somebody else bothered to make a difference in ours. "Bother it Forward" can describe this phenomenon. And combining this all with humor and laughter shared, as Captain Perry suggests, is powerful indeed.

Epilogue

I was inspired to embark on this project by my experience of being part of a supportive community that fostered life-changing benefits. With my perspective as a psychologist, gym owner, coach, athlete, and mom, I am keenly interested in the power of a group of individuals sharing a common, positive goal. The personal stories I have gathered for this project have furthered, enriched, and reinforced my belief in the power of community. While CrossFit isn't the only example of a community driving people toward excellence and self-improvement, it is the one I know most intimately and the one that has changed my life.

CrossFit has evolved organically from being a great workout offering great results, to becoming a powerhouse community fueled by relationships born of shared challenges and mutual respect. The CrossFit program continues to motivate a vast network of members of all ages, at all levels of fitness and ability. The future of CrossFit and its mission to change the face of fitness lies not only in the adult population but also with the children and teens who are actively involved. CrossFit Kids extends the reach of the program and its community to young people worldwide. The benefits of the workouts, the family atmosphere of kids having fun, with friends, parents, and coaches cheering them on, are inspiring and significant. Children learn that hard work, physical challenge, and persistence, combined with the pleasures of camaraderie and altruism, can make a real difference in their lives and in the world around them.

In interviewing the individuals whose stories appear here, I have been humbled and awe-struck by their courage, generosity, and accomplishments. My hope is that you have been inspired by the narratives of ordinary people doing extraordinary things with their time and energy, with mind and body, and with the resources they have to share. Perhaps you will find it within yourself to take in the power of a community and make positive changes in your life. Or perhaps you will take the inspiration a step further and start a community of your own, based on a shared interest or goal, in order to better the lives of the members of the group. Perhaps you will "bother it forward." When you have a group of people supporting you, the landscape is limitless and the possibilities endless.

NOTES

1. *CrossFit Training Guide*. CrossFit, Inc., p.5. http://www.crossfit.com/cf-seminars/CertRefs/CF_Manual_v4.pdf

2. D. W. Winnicott, "The Theory of the Parent-Infant Relationship," in *The Maturational Processes and the Facilitating Environment: Studies in the Theory of Emotional Development* (New York: International Universities Press, 1965), pp. 37–55.

3. Hillary Clinton, *It Takes a Village to Raise A Child: And Other Lessons Children Teach Us* (New York: Simon and Schuster, 1996), pp. 11–12.

4. Francis Fukuyama, *The Great Disruption: Human Nature and the Reconstitution of Social Order* (New York: The Free Press, New York, 1999), pp. 278–79.

5. Robert Putnam, *Bowling Alone* (New York: Simon and Schuster, 2000), p. 19.

6. L. J. Hanifan, "The Rural School Community Center," *Annals of the American Academy of Political and Social Science* 67: 130.

7. Putnam, *Bowling*, p. 296.

8. Emile Durkheim, *Suicide: A Study in Sociology* (New York: The Free Press, 1951), p. 209.

9. Durkheim, *Suicide*, pp. 209–10.

10. Lisa Berkman and S. Leonard Syme, "Social Networks, Host Resistance, and Mortality: A Nine-Year Follow-Up Study of Alameda County Residents," *American Journal of Epidemiology* 109, no. 2 (1970): 186–204.

11. C. H. Kroenke, L. D. Kubzansky, E. S. Schernhammer, M. D. Holmes, and I. Kawachi, "Social Networks, Social Support, and Survival after Breast Cancer Diagnosis," *Journal of Clinical Oncology* 24, no. 7 (2006): 1105–11; Y. L. Michael, L. F.

Berkman, G. A. Colditz, M. D. Holmes, and I. Kawachi, "Social Networks and Health-Related Quality of Life in Breast Cancer Survivors: A Prospective Study," *Journal of Psychosomatic Research* 52, no. 5 (2002): 285–93.

12. K. Kiewra, "The Science of Resiliency," *FOCUS: News from Harvard Medical, Dental and Public Health Schools*. http://www.focushms.com/features/the-science-of-resiliency

13. Lisa F. Berkman, "The Role of Social Relations in Health Promotion," *Psychosomatic Medicine*.57, no. 3 (1995): 245–54; R. S. Baron, C. E. Cutrona, D. Hicklin, et al., "Social Support and Immune Function among Spouses of Cancer Patients," Journal of Personality and Social Psychology 59 (1990): 344–52; R. W. Bartrop, E. Luckhurst, L. Lazarus, et al., "Depressed Lymphocyte Function after Bereavement," Lancet 1 (1977): 834–36.

14. Putnam, Bowling, p. 331.

15. K. Viswanath, W. R. Steele, and J. R. Finnegan Jr., "Social Capital and Health: Civic Engagement, Community Size, and Recall of Health Messages," *American Journal of Public Health* 96 no. 8 (2006): 1456–61.

16. Mark K. Smith, "Community," in *Encyclopedia of Informal Education*, http://www.infed.org/community/community.htm.

17. Zygmunt Bauman, *Community: Seeking Safety in an Insecure World* (Cambridge, UK: Polity Press, 2001), p. 149.

18. Greg Glassman, Community Support: An Interview with *Fast Company* magazine, *CrossFit Journal*, October 2, 2011, http://library.crossfit.com/free/video/CFJ_WhatIsCrossFitGregGlassman_CommunitySupport.mov

19. Matt Ridley, *The Origins of Virtue* (New York: Penguin, 1997), p. 249.

20. Fukuyama, *The Great Disruption*, p. 155.

21. Hanifan, "The Rural School," p. 130.

22. Elizabeth Frazer, *The Problem of Communitarian Politics: Unity and Conflict* (Oxford: Oxford University Press, 1999), p. 83.

23. L. F. Berkman, T. Glass, I. Brissett, and T. E. Seeman, "From Social Integration to Health: Durkheim in the New Millennium,"

Social Science and Medicine 51 (2000): 849.

24. V. R. Waldron and S. C. Yungbluth, "Assessing Student Outcomes in Communication-Intensive Learning Communities: A Two-Year Longitudinal Study of Academic Performance and Retention," *Southern Communication Journal* 72, no. 3 (2007): 285–302.

25. W. J. Bauer, "Public Perceptions and the Importance of Community: Observations from a California Indian Who Has Lived, Learned, and Taught in Indiana, Oklahoma, and Wyoming," *The American Indian Quarterly* 27, nos. 1–2 (2003): 62–66.

26. Bauman, *Community*, p.2.

27. Putnam, *Bowling*, p. 21.

28. Alejandro Portes, Social Capital: Its Origins and Applications in Modern Sociology, *Annual Review of Sociology* 24 (1998): 18.

29. Ibid., p. 17.

30. Bauman, *Community*, p. 121.

31. Seth Godin, *Seth Godin's Blog*, http://sethgodin.typepad.com

32. D. Hirsch, "Report Ranks Camden Most Dangerous U.S. City," *Courier-Post*, November 24.

33. Steve Liberati, www.stevesclub.org

34. Seth Godin, *Tribes: We Need You to Lead Us* (New York: Penguin, 2008).

35. Ibid., p. 9.

36. Olivia Smith, "Working Out Together Lightens the Load," *Redwood Bark Online*, January 28, http://redwoodbark.org/index.php?option=com_content&task=view&id=2356&Itemid=5

37. William Shakespeare, *Henry V*, Act 4, scene 3, line 60.

38. Carey Peterson, "The Disposable Heroes Project: Part 4," *CrossFit Journal*, http://journal.crossfit.com/2010/05/brad-100-mile-4.tpl

39. W. N. Burton, C. Chen, D. J. Conti, A. B. Schultz, G. Pransky, and D. W. Edington, "The Association of Health Risks with On-the-Job Productivity, *Journal of Occupational and Environmental Medicine* 47, no. 8 (2005): 769–77; W. N. Burton, K. T. McCallister, C. Chen, and D. W. Edington, "The Association

of Health Status, Worksite Fitness Center Participation, and Two Measures of Productivity," *Journal of Occupational and Environmental Medicine* 47, no. 4 (2005): 343–51; D. M. Gates, P. Succop, B. J. Brehm, G. L. Gillespie, and B. D. Somners, "Obesity and Presenteeism: The Impact of Body Mass Index on Workplace Productivity," *Journal of Occupational and Environmental Medicine* 50, no. 1 (2008): 39–45.

40. J. Leutzinger and D. Blanke, "The Effect of a Corporate Fitness Program on Perceived Worker Productivity," *Journal of Health, Behavior, Education, & Promotion* 15, no. 5(1991): 20–29; R. L. Bertera, "The Effects of Workplace Health Promotion on Absenteeism and Employment Costs in a Large Industrial Population," *American Journal of Public Health* 80 no. 9 (1990): 1101–5; R. J. Ozminkowski, R. L. Dunn, R. Z. Goetzel, R. I. Cantor, J. Murnane, and M. Harrison, "A Return on Investment Evaluation of the Citibank, N.A., Health Management Program," *American Journal of Public Health* 14, no. 1, (1999): 31–43; D. Hillier, F. Fewell, W. Cann, and V. Shephard, "Wellness at Work: Enhancing the Quality of Our Working Lives," *Journal of Occupational and Environmental Medicine* 17, no. 5 (2005): 419–31.

41. John J. Ratey, *Spark: The Revolutionary New Science of Exercise and the Brain* (New York: Little, Brown, 2008).

42. Allison Belger, "CrossFit after 40," *CrossFit Journal*. http://journal.crossfit.com/2010/01/masters-athletes.tpl

43. Greg Glassman, "Community Support: An Interview with *Fast Company* magazine, October 2, 2011, http://journal.crossfit.com/2011/10/greggamescommunitysupport.tpl

About the Author

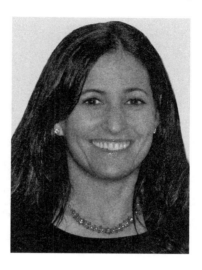

As co-owner of four CrossFit affiliate gyms, Allison Belger juggles management of the family business, her work as a licensed psychologist and fitness coach, and her role as mom to two young daughters. She knows firsthand the importance of community—of having a network of mutual support and human connection in the midst of our hectic, technology-driven lives. A former division-one collegiate soccer player and five-time marathoner, she has also been part of the wilderness adventure community and has trained for various elite athletic events, competing both individually and as part of a team.

Allison earned a BA from Dartmouth College, a Master's Degree from Northwestern University, and a Doctorate in Clinical Psychology from the Wright Institute in Berkeley, California.